The Invisible TRAUMA

Coping with PTSD

DAVE MORGAN

First published 2022

Big Sky Publishing Pty Ltd
PO Box 303, Newport, NSW 2106, Australia
Phone: 1300 364 611
Fax: (61 2) 9918 2396
Email: info@bigskypublishing.com.au
Web: www.bigskypublishing.com.au

Cover design and typesetting: Think Productions

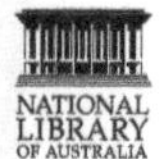

A catalogue record for this book is available from the National Library of Australia

Title: The Invisible Trauma. Coping with PTSD
ISBN: 9781922765345

Printed and bound in Australia by Griffin Press

The Invisible TRAUMA

Coping with PTSD

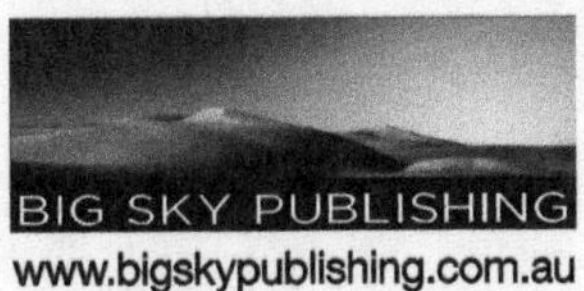

www.bigskypublishing.com.au

DAVE MORGAN

I stand alone in silent darkness
Screaming out aloud
From another frightening and terrifying nightmare
With my body shaking and sweating in terror
Wondering
'Why Me?'
and
'Why Wars?'
With no answers

Dave Morgan

CONTENTS

THE WRAITH WITH THE FOUR LETTER NAME

In darkest night there comes a wraith to knock upon your door,
clad in tattered, twisted memories of a time you lived before.
It demands you open up that door and expose a wounded soul,
to live once more that nightmare time that nothing can console.

That wraith that others cannot see controls your tortured mind.
Its evil garb of times of war, by your demons … well designed.
It wraps you with that dreaded shroud 'til scarce your breath will come
'til tight your heart, so wet your sweat, until your screams succumb.

Then finally clad in such mawkish garb it leaves you in dawn's light,
a light that brings no comfort from those memories … No respite.
You live your day's life clothed like that wraith, tattered, twisted, bare,
to wait in fear for coming nights, full knowing who'll be there.

This wraith that comes now has a name … Four letters … Christened fear.
It's not only yours, it knows many more, and it won't just visit here.
It knows your mates, those ones who've suffered, and others that still do.
And though it feels like yours alone, it haunts many more than you.

A single twig is not hard to break but if you bind a few together,
A bond like this will confuse the wraith, those garments will cease to tether.
PTSD, that dark night wraith, must never own your soul.
Discard that shroud of darker times and let this new time make you whole.

ACKNOWLEDGEMENTS

I want to thank a few special people for their support.

David Murphy, a mate who served with me in Vietnam, contributed one of the 'Forewords' and edited the book. David has a wealth of experience editing other veterans' stories. His help was invaluable, and I believe I could not have completed my story without him.

I feel overwhelmed with the contributions of three doctors to the 'Foreword' section. A special thank you to Dr Michael Naughton – SMO Australian Army Force Vietnam (1965-66) and CO 1st Australian Field Hospital (1969-70) – whom I met at a GMRF breakfast seminar for veterans' sleep therapy study in 2019; to Dr Justine Evans – Clinical Psychologist GMRF – whom I met while attending a PTSD Programme at Greenslopes Private Hospital in 2015; and Dr Paul Cadzow, my Consultant Psychiatrist since 2009. I am very grateful for the effort and research Dr Sarah Hampton at GMRF put into her very clear explanation of CBT-I and IRT therapies and the benefits they offer sleep disorders. Her work appears in Chapter 29.

A special thank you to Graham McLoughlin, a very gifted poet and singer for contributing a poem which really hits the spot.

Also, thanks to the veterans for their contributions. I am profoundly grateful to Maureen Bronjes (MOZ) – we met at Cooinda Mental Health Service PTSD programme; Andy Fermo – I did a podcast for him on 'Invisible Injuries'; Ian Fraser – Dawson River Retreat; Michelle Fraser (daughter of Ian) – Dawson River Retreat; and Jeanette Holland – Cooinda Mental Health Service PTSD programme. Their personal stories – 'My Experience' – on PTSD, added extra depth to my account of PTSD. I know it was not easy to write about your traumas and issues, so I admire you all.

My children, Michelle and David have been coping all their lives with my PTSD. They have now written here about how they've been affected by it. My pride in them can't be put into words.

Finally, my wife, Debbie, has been my life-support for so many years. It was great that she was able to contribute 'The Last Word'.

Dave Morgan

Sunshine Coast, Queensland

2022

FOREWORD

Dr Michael Naughton,

SMO Australian Army Force Vietnam 1965-66
and CO 1st Australian Field Hospital 1969-70

In any war the health of a fit soldier can drastically change in an instant and so it was for the men and women in the Vietnam war. While the consequences of major physical injury from a high velocity gunshot wound or from shrapnel from an exploding anti-personnel mine or from the explosive effects of an artillery shell or mortar were obvious, the effects of psychological injury were not.

Adverse psychological effects resulting from war have been known for many years and labels such as Shell Shock or Battle Fatigue were applied. However since the Vietnam experience and subsequent research, those adverse psychological effects are now known as Post Traumatic Stress Disorder. PTSD can result from experiencing a near death incident, or the violent injury or death of a mate or from treating the major wounds of battle casualties. A high percentage recover from the acute effects of psychological injury but for many, the experience may be the start of a chronic disorder that can affect the well-being of sufferers for the remainder of their lives.

In Vietnam there was a concentrated effort to save the lives of battle casualties. First aid in the field and rapid evacuation by helicopter to sophisticated medical facilities was a major factor in the survival of many battle casualties who would not have survived in previous conflicts. The helicopter ambulance provided smooth and rapid transport so that a casualty could arrive at a surgical facility in a matter of hours and in some cases in only one hour. The medical teams were primarily involved in saving life and restoring the highest level of function that the wounds allowed. The medical services in Vietnam were also heavily engaged with the management of tropical diseases especially malaria which was causing significant loss of manpower.

What was not obvious and possibly more sinister was the impact of the psychological injury incurred not only by the wounded battle casualties but by men and women who were not physically injured. However, the impact of psychological injury was not neglected. The Walter Reid Army Institute Research, Vietnam was stationed in Saigon and was actively involved in research of diseases encountered by American troops in Vietnam. One of the Walter Reid researchers was Dr Peter Bourne[1] who studied the psychological and physiological effects of combat stress. In 1966 he was invited to visit 1st Battalion Royal Australian Regiment, 1RAR to study the psychological health

1 Bourne, P. *Men, Stress and Vietnam.* Little Brown, Boston 1969. Bourne, P (ed) *Psychology and Physiology of Stress*, Academic Press, New York 1970

of our troops. He readily agreed to our request and stayed for a short time. 1RAR was coming to the end of its tour of duty and there was obvious evidence of physical fatigue and the "wind-down syndrome" but the psychological health of the unit and the morale was high. Army commanders have always been concerned about the effects of the morale of units under command and good morale was considered essential for a fighting force to be effective in its mission.

In the years following, an Australian psychiatrist was available to our troops. These psychiatrists were private practitioners but were also members of the Army Reserve and volunteered for 3 months service at 1st Australian Field Hospital stationed at Vung Tau. The psychiatrists visited 1st Australian Task Force which was located at Nui Dat to gauge the psychological well-being of the soldiers. They also conducted individual consultations with men and women referred by Army medical officers who were posted to front line and supporting logistical units. The number with psychological problems was small and no obvious trends in trauma-related psychological injury were observed.

But Post Traumatic Stress Disorder has now emerged as a major problem effecting both veteran and civilian communities. First it was seen in Vietnam veterans but now it has been recognized in more recent conflicts in Somalia, Iraq, Afghanistan and in military interventions such as the Rwanda genocide or from natural disasters such as the Indian Ocean tsunami.

Many Vietnam veterans returning to Australia did not receive a warm welcome home. There were of course memories of trade union bans disrupting delivery of mail and essential supplies and in Vietnam the troops took action to ridicule those responsible by printing "Punch a Postie" and "Wallop a Wharfie" slogans on envelopes of homeward bound mail. Much worse, on return to Australia there were the anti-War Demonstrations in which even a few politicians participated. Some veterans even suffered personal insults such as being spat on or being reviled as 'baby burners". A veteran Army nurse tearfully reported that protestors assembled outside a military hospital and abused the men recovering from the effects of their wounds. In one case the staff and patients of a military hospital had to be evacuated because of a viable bomb threat.

Incidents such as these caused anger and dismay to veterans and may have added to the psychological stress already present.

In his book "The Invisible Trauma" Dave Morgan gives a detailed and clear account of his battle with PTSD. He describes his traumatic experience in Vietnam and how PTSD gradually emerged after his return to Australia. He experienced negative thinking, confusion, intense anger, alcohol abuse, and thoughts of suicide. This caused great distress. He expresses his experience frankly and opens a window to understanding the problems of a man suffering from PTSD.

Remarkably, he commenced a long and successful career with the Bureau of Meteorology and he progressed through the ranks while all the time forced to deal with problems which he struggled to contain. His accounts of life at Giles in the remote Gibson Desert and later experiences with the ANARE Meteorology program, first on Macquarie Island (as Officer-in-Charge) and then Davis Base Antarctica, are wonderful and exciting. His ambition to work at Casey Base Antarctica was finally in his grasp but ended suddenly when he suffered a head injury and brain trauma. This ended his career with the Bureau of Meteorology.

So finally, after 40 years of suffering, he sought treatment for his PTSD. In this he was lovingly supported by his wife and family, a support often denied veterans whose relationships do not survive the domestic upheaval caused by PTSD.

I first met Dave in 2019 at a meeting sponsored by the Gallipoli Research Foundation at Greenslopes Hospital which was chaired by Professor John Pearn, a colleague from our shared service at 1st Australian Field Hospital. The Gallipoli Research Foundation and the Returned and Services League (Queensland Branch) have established project "PTSD Initiative" which provides support to veterans and which Dave as a participant describes in this book.

I was impressed by Dave's account of his long fight with PTSD. I am also impressed by his writings and his willingness to assist fellow veterans. In this he has made a valuable contribution and his book is well worth a read by those who are interested in this chronic disorder.

There is no completely effective treatment for PTSD, but people like Dave Morgan are doing all they can to reach that goal.

FOREWORD

DAVID MURPHY,

RADIO OPERATOR 104 SIG SQN 1969

PTSD is a debilitating mental illness which has been around forever but only relatively recently been seriously tackled because of its prevalence among Vietnam veterans. There has always been a general reluctance for anyone with mental illness to parade it publicly – who, after all, wants to be tagged a "loonie" or "weak in the pants"? – but veterans can take credit for persisting in demanding proper treatment. Some, like Dave Morgan, have taken the battle a step further by exposing their personal traumas in an effort to help others.

Military conflict is an ugly, dangerous, deadly activity generally carried out on a grand scale so it is easy to forget that many individuals have to do the dirty work. Those individuals can't exactly "down tools" and get on with life in society when the war is over, yet Vietnam veterans were expected to do just that.

I was one of them, a Nasho just 15 months out of a seminary when I boarded a jet for Vietnam with Dave in early January 1969. The government allowed others like me to return early to Australia for Christmas but Regular soldiers like Dave had to complete their full 365 days there. Cruel? I think so.

The worst cruelty, though, was the government's assurance to Nashos that we would be able to take back our lives after 2 years as though nothing had happened in that interval – sort of "hold your breath and it's gone"! Well, plenty had happened; all of us had been through the ultimate life-changing experience.

Governments are often prone to make promises they don't keep. This was one of them. We were used, abused and then, job done, refused assistance when we sought help. Veterans came home to find themselves unwelcome, ostracised and alienated by a vocal anti-war minority. It is said that those who stay silent in the face of wrong are equally guilty of committing that wrong. Veterans took that on board.

Unable to discuss our problems, blocked from any help with them, we locked them away where they festered and grew as you will see in Dave's account. 50 years on, I know of veterans on acreages west of Bundaberg (probably in many places around Australia) who are still at war, living isolated lives, surrounded by trenches, barbed wire and booby traps and keeping automatic assault rifles at hand. What an indictment on the nation that is!

Don't expect this book to be PTSD 101. If you're looking for something like that, you'll need to search the medical literature – there's plenty to choose from there. This is a very painful, personal account of an individual intent on self-medicating, believing his difficulties are his alone and therefore, his to overcome. It's a book for all those suffering similarly, not solely veterans either. You will see yourself on every page.

Morg has put himself through agony recording many painful examples of the difficulties posed by his condition. By detailing his treatments, he offers hope to fellow sufferers and encouragement for them to seek professional help.

A real soldier would never leave a mate behind on the battlefield. Morg is still doing his best to bring his mates home.

POST-TRAUMATIC STRESS DISORDER

Dr Paul Cadzow
Consultant Psychiatrist

Post-Traumatic Stress Disorder has been Dave's companion for decades. I say companion because although it has been a significant part of most of his adult life, it hasn't defined him and Dave has lived a life characterised by loving family relationships, intellectual curiosity, commitment to helping others and an interesting career. Some of those life experiences, specifically the pursuit of a career that led to him living and working in isolated, environmentally extreme places like Antarctica, he attributes to his adaptations to living with PTSD.

In one sense, it is not possible to live a full-life without experiencing losses and exposure to potentially traumatising experiences. Not all experiences like this however lead to problematic stress reactions or proceed on to the development of Post-Traumatic Stress Disorder. Indeed, two-thirds of people exposed to traumatic events will not develop PTSD. Both the nature of the incident and personal characteristics of the individual can contribute to the development of PTSD. PTSD is mostly often associated with military service, but occurs in emergency personnel, civilians and in response to both man-made and natural disasters. For military veterans, around 8% will experience PTSD throughout their lives and 5% are likely to have PTSD at any time.

One of the important things to understand is that PTSD, although distressing, is a treatable condition. There are a range of possible treatments and Dave has had many of these. Trauma-focussed cognitive behavioural therapy (TF-CBT), describes treatments that employs the principles of CBT with some form of trauma processing. Generally, TF-CBT includes components of exposure therapy, including imaginal exposure[2] and graded in vivo exposure[3].

When Dave was first being treated for his PTSD, he underwent a treatment course of TF-CBT with prolonged exposure. This produced a reduction of his symptoms for some years. He has subsequently done a CBT-based group trauma program. The work of processing traumatic experiences can be challenging and exhausting, and this was certainly Dave's experience. On one occasion, he travelled home from his session feeling completely exhausted and having to lie down in the back of the car. The taxi driver had to assist him into his house. But the benefit of doing it is a reduction in symptoms

2 imagining feared images or situations

3 Directly facing a feared object, situation or activity in real life. For example, someone with a fear of snakes might be instructed to handle a snake, or someone with social anxiety might be instructed to give a speech in front of an audience.

and in Dave's case there was a clear objective evidence of this because he tracks the frequency of his nightmares and was able to see a reduction in them after the treatment course.

VALUE OF DAVE MORGAN'S PTSD INSIGHTS

Dr Justine Evans
Clinical Psychologist
Gallipoli Medical Research Foundation

I have had the privilege of meeting Dave Morgan on multiple occasions in my work as a Clinical Psychologist at Greenslopes Private Hospital and at the Gallipoli Medical Research Foundation.

Dave has always been generous with his time and willingness to share his personal experiences of living with posttraumatic stress disorder (PTSD). In this book (particularly the chapter on PTSD Programs and Challenges) Dave provides incredibly beneficial information on his experiences of treatment through the lens of someone who has lived with PTSD since the Vietnam War.

It provides an honest and hopeful account of the benefits he has experienced through his long-term commitment to psychological treatment. Last year, Dave agreed to talk at a Breakfast Seminar supporting GMRF's Veteran Sleep Therapy study about the impact that nightmares have had on his sleep. Dave's willingness to do this speaks to his bravery and generosity in sharing his story for others' benefit and his belief in the potential for improvements to be made through high-quality research.

INTRODUCTION

How does taking a trip down memory lane make you feel?

Your memories are a part of you, reflections of the adventures you've had, the choices you've made, the lives you've touched. Memories should not feel like a prison. Sadly, it only takes one moment, one awful memory, to cause a lifetime of suffering.

I am 73 years old, served in Vietnam for 366 days, and have spent the last fifty-two years (18,993 days to 7th January 2022) suffering from the experience as a result of severe post-traumatic stress disorder (PTSD). My aim is to share my story with the hope of shining a light on this devastating condition for the benefit of younger veterans and anyone who suffers from PTSD.

What is PTSD?

PTSD, or post-traumatic stress disorder is a set of reactions that can occur after someone has experienced a traumatic event. About two thirds of Australians will experience at least one traumatic event in their lives such as a car crash, fires, mining tragedies, air and maritime disasters, floods or earthquakes, domestic violence, robberies, rape and wars.

After a traumatic experience most people will develop an acute stress reaction such as feeling frightened, sad and disconnected for a few weeks but after about a month they come to terms with it and their stress reactions dissipate. However, for some people like me, these symptoms never go away.

The main symptoms of PTSD are as follows:

- Re-living the traumatic event through distressing, unwanted memories, vivid nightmares, and flashbacks. This can also include feeling terribly upset or having intense physical reactions such as heart palpitations or being unable to breathe, hyper-ventilating, nausea, sweating and muscle tension when reminded of the traumatic event.
- Avoiding reminders of the traumatic event, including activities, places, people, conversations, thoughts, or feelings that bring back distressing memories of the trauma.
- Negative thoughts and feelings such as fear, anger, guilt, or feeling flat or numb. Distorted thinking about the causes or consequences and blaming themselves or others for what happened during or after the traumatic event, feeling cut off from friends and family, and losing interest in day-to-day activities.
- Feeling overly alert and wound up, causing trouble sleeping or concentrating, feeling angry or irritable, taking risks or indulging in self-destructive behaviour, being easily startled or being constantly on the lookout for danger.

People with PTSD also experience other mental health problems like depression and anxiety and some may look to using alcohol or drugs as a way of coping.

Over the years PTSD impacted every aspect of my life, made it difficult to function normally at work, at home and socially. It also affected my own family's lives. I couldn't sleep for more than two hours a night, I drank heavily at times, I would quickly lose my temper, or spiral back into depression and begin contemplating suicide.

As a Vietnam war veteran there was no less PTSD at the end of the Vietnam War than there would have been at the end of the First World War. It was then known as 'shell shock', and in the Second World War as 'battle fatigue'. When I first sought help from a doctor in the mid-1970s, the term 'posttraumatic stress disorder' did not exist. The doctor diagnosed me with severe 'war depression', gave me medication and sent me on my way. There was no recognition of the extent of my suffering, no treatment options, no help at all. I was alone.

Something I've always struggled with is the question 'why me?' Why did I get this horrible thing when other people who experienced trauma didn't?

Maybe I was vulnerable to PTSD from the earlier days in my life or was it in my DNA at birth?

CHAPTER 1

MY EARLY YEARS

I was born on the 4th of March 1948, in South Yarra, Melbourne, a fashionable seven minutes after my twin brother, Don. We were the new additions to a family which included two other children – an older brother Gerald George who was 10 years of age and my sister Sybil Patricia, who was 8 at the time of our arrival. On September 9, 1947 – just after Mum, Sybella fell pregnant with Don and I, my father Gerald Augustine Morgan known as Gus, died unexpectedly. He was in the Merchant Navy for most of his life and served during the Second World War and I wouldn't be surprised if he had PTSD as he had been a heavy smoker and drinker. I know my Mum suffered from depression, due to not only losing her husband that day, but the inheritance she'd invested in the family café business in Alice Springs after the War vanished with him. With no money and no income, my Mum single-handedly became the backbone of the family, shifting around different States to find work to support her young family. All this uncertainty, pressure and struggle caught up with her, causing depression.

Being a twin is special in my mind. We were identical, and no one could tell us apart. We got used to being called by each other's name. Growing up we often teased our Mum about getting us mixed up when we were born, but as a mother she knew the difference. We were both born with red hair and blue eyes. Apparently, the difference was I had a chubby face compared to Don. I slept more while he was wider awake, active and alert. We were close in every way. Mum had to be careful to treat us the same; if not, one of us would get upset. We played together, laughed together, cried together, shared our friends together, and felt each other's pain together.

Don was the boss, leader and more dominant than me, but I did not mind, I just followed him. He was always there for me. I remember when I was going home from school in Echuca one day when an aborigine boy started pushing and hitting me. Don jumped in and protected me and wrestled the aborigine boy to the ground causing him to run off. There were times when both of us got into trouble from Mum, but we always defended each other.

At school Don was more academic than me; he wanted to learn about things and study while I struggled and hated school. I was more of a dreamer. As we got older, we became more competitive with each other in the backyard, playing football, cricket or tennis. I think this started with me as I felt he was better than me at school, so I would try to outperform and beat him in the backyard. It did not work as he was just as determined as me to win. This caused a lot of heated fights, with poor Mum having to break them up.

My days growing up were the happiest days of my life, full of adventures, with my fondest memory being freedom. We were free to roam anywhere for adventure, like to a mate's place, to the river or creek to go fishing, to the beach and to ride our bikes anywhere. Back then there was hardly any crime. People trusted each other, leaving house doors open and unlocked or leaving car windows down with the keys in the ignition or leaving a bike on the side path. Like all young kids I experienced different incidents like stitches in deep cuts, crushed fingers, haemorrhage after getting my tonsils out and a broken wrist.

At the time all the above incidents caused some stress and fear for me. I crushed my fingers by accidentally putting my left fingers in one of the swinging doors in the dining car on the Ghan train from Alice Springs to Adelaide. Two fingers were crushed so badly that the train conductors were considering a rendezvous with the Flying Doctor at the next siding. However, as luck would have it, there was a doctor on board the train and he stabilised the injury until we got back to civilisation in Adelaide. Two painful days later, my fingers had become infected. Mum took me straight to the Adelaide hospital where their first concern was that one or two of the fingers might need to be amputated. Fortunately, after a week of treatment at the hospital with antibiotics I was given the all clear by the doctor.

During the winters of Grade 3 and 4 at Echuca State School, Don and I came down with tonsillitis. Our family doctor, who did house calls, saw it as an ongoing problem and decided that our tonsils must come out. He booked Don and I into the hospital, with our operations scheduled for a month apart. As Don was older by those all-important seven minutes, he was set to face the operation first. Off he went bravely, apparently making good use of his 7 extra minutes of maturity and the operation was successful.

When my turn came, I was not as cooperative as Mum and the nursing staff would have liked. Understandably, I was scared. Mum took me to the hospital via taxi. At 6am, she tried to drop me off, but I stubbornly refused to go into the building. The old matron, in her sixties, tried to coax me inside but the thought of what awaited me there persuaded me to stand my ground. Having had no luck enticing me, dragging me in was the next strategy employed. I was small but agile and managed to get away. I ran for my life with the matron and the nurses chasing me up the driveway. It would have been an amusing sight I suppose, but at the time I was desperately bent on self-preservation and for me, there was no humour involved. They eventually caught me and got me back to the hospital where I had my operation later that morning.

The operation was pronounced successful and for the next two days I had ice cream and jelly. When the time came to go home, Mum arrived in the taxi. With my pride a little wounded from being forced to have my tonsils out, I refused to go home in the taxi and instead, I challenged Mum to a race home, her in the taxi and me running. I did not give her the chance to refuse and I dashed off in the direction of home. Admirably, I made it in good enough time to beat the taxi, but it was all too short a victory as about half an hour later, I started vomiting blood in a bucket. The family doctor had to come out to see me again. Back I went to hospital, spending 2 days in the intensive care ward. When I was released into Mum's care at the end of that second stay, you can believe that I peacefully took the taxi home with her.

The broken wrist incident happened in my third year at Echuca High school when I performed gym work on a monkey bar. I was excellent on the bar, probably due to my light weight. The boys in my group had a competition to see who could swing and jump along the bar the furthest. I was leading the competition until my last try. My hands slipped off the bar and I fell. I landed on my back with my left hand bent up under me. I was winded badly and I could hardly get my breath. That was the least of my worries when I looked down, shocked to see a bone jutting out from my left wrist. The headmaster rushed me to the Echuca hospital. After painkillers and X-rays, the hospital surgeon decided to reset my wrist bone. They put me under anaesthetic late in the afternoon and I came out of it early in the evening with my left wrist and arm in plaster.

But nothing compared to one incident which still haunts and angers me to this day.

Back in my school days in Echuca in the early sixties, I usually walked to school. There was a little special needs girl who lived in the Housing Commission Home just around the corner from our house. She was a couple of years younger than me. She used to get teased quite a lot. This morning, a group of boys and girls had been teasing her when I came across her. The kids had just run away, and I saw her crying, so I stopped and asked her if she was okay.

That was precisely the moment when a well-to-do gentleman who owned one of the local garages came out of his house. He was wearing his dressing gown. He had heard the commotion and saw the little girl crying and screaming and me standing there with her. You can imagine what happened. He put 2 and 2 together and got 5. He assumed that I was the one who had made her cry by teasing her. He yelled out to me. He shouted at me to stop teasing the little girl and come over to him. He wanted to talk to me, he said.

As the saying goes, 'If you have nothing to hide…', so I did as he said. As soon as I moved within his grasp, he grabbed me and shook me. "I am sick of you kids teasing this girl," he yelled. I naturally defended myself telling him that it was the other kids. He didn't believe me. Summarily tried and found guilty, he dragged me roughly by the arms and neck, forcing me into the laundry of his house. In his robes, not robes of office, but a bathrobe, he had judged me. It was extremely humiliating and frightening. His wife appeared at the back door and he told her that he had finally caught up with one of the kids who always teased that poor little girl.

He instructed his wife to get his clothes ready as he was going to take 'the brat' into the headmaster to let him deal out an appropriate punishment. He then locked me in the laundry. By this time, I was shaking and confused. He got ready and collected me, none too gently for a gentleman. He put me in his car. The entire trip to school was spent with me trying to explain the truth, to no avail.

At school, the headmaster and the 'gentleman' discussed the matter. The gentleman made it clear that he wanted me punished.

I pleaded my innocence to the headmaster but again without success. The headmaster was fuming. My punishment was 8 of the best – four cuts on each hand while the so-called gentleman looked on. I had to bear the undeserved lashes without any buffer. It hurt more than my hands. My pride, my sense of justice and my respect were hurt more.

At lunchtime I went home, I was so upset and shaken as I told my Mum the whole story. She was outraged that this could happen to me. She went to see the headmaster on my behalf but not even she could shake his conviction that I had done it. It is a terrible thing to be disbelieved. It took me a while to get over the whole incident. If it hadn't been for Mum's support and belief in me, I don't know how I would have moved past the event. I felt a lasting sense of bitterness that the headmaster immediately and irrevocably believed a well-to-do adult over an earnest – and don't forget – innocent, poor kid.

> ***I look back on my life and say, "Yes that definitely is a PTSD symptom from a stressful event".***
>
> ***Years later when I first joined the Army I'd go to Echuca on leave and often walked by the house, hoping to front this so-called gentleman but I never did. Just as well because I know I would have been up for a serious assault charge.***

Due to Mum's health and looking for work, we lived in a lot of places when I was growing up including Somers in Victoria, Mildura in Victoria, Alice Springs in the Northern Territory, on a farm near Balaclava in South Australia, Launceston in Tasmania, Echuca back in Victoria, and finally Caloundra on the Sunshine Coast in Queensland.

Mum suffered from chronic bronchitis and her doctor advised her to move to Queensland where the warmer climate would improve her health. Mum sought help from Legacy, an organisation that helps dependents of deceased Australian service men and women who served during wars. Legacy found us a house in Caloundra, where we discovered Caloundra was the perfect place to live, not only for Mum's health but for Don and I, our final school years plus a lifestyle of sun, surf and sand.

It wasn't all about fun and games as I soon got a job working on a milk run on weekends plus public holidays. I managed to put some money away over two years with the job. Don and I also got jobs as postmen for the Christmas/New Year holiday breaks. After gaining our Junior Certificate, Don and I decided to keep going at school to complete our Sub-Senior year or grade eleven. One of my teachers was an officer in the Citizens Military Force (CMF) at Nambour 9 RQR (Royal Queensland Regiment) and he got me interested in joining. I enlisted in the CMF on the 14th April 1966 at Nambour. My Army number, 123256, was easy to remember – the 2nd 2 was half the 4 in the number sequence. My commitments to the CMF included a weekly parade at the drill hall, and one weekend a month. I enjoyed every moment. The whole experience held newfound adventure for me. So much so, that I began to think I might like to join the Regular Army. I was getting just average marks in Sub-Senior, so I decided it would be my last year at school. I loved the sound and sight of an aircraft. I'd always wanted to fly since the day in my first year of primary school when a biplane came down in a paddock at Somers and all the kids went running out to see it. So I was thinking of trying to pursue a career in either the Army or as a pilot.

I decided to take some flying lessons, so Mum contacted a flying school at Maroochydore airport, Sunland Aviation. Three times a week I took a one-hour lesson, eventually flying solo. I would've kept going indefinitely but money I had saved, or rather the lack of it, had become a challenge. After a request to Legacy for help to continue with lessons was denied, I applied to join the Regular Army hoping to get into their aviation program indirectly.

While learning to fly I had two incidents when flying solo. The first happened when returning to the airport from the training area, I entered a large cumulus cloud at four thousand feet and experienced a total white out with strong winds and heavy rain. I panicked and immediately descended. Without completing proper circuit and landing procedure, I overshot the dirt runway and landed in a soft grassy area. My flying instructor was not amused and gave me a tongue-lashing.

The second incident happened when I descended to 200 feet in the 'Cessna 150' and flew along the long stretch of Peregian surf beach practising forced landings. I got that fun idea from a young farmer who was learning to fly at the same time as me, but our fun act apparently upset the local surf fishermen who complained to the police. Once again, I got a tongue lashing from my instructor telling me and the young farmer we were on our last chance and were only to practise forced landings in the training area north of the airport.

All up my total hours with flying instructor Kevin Henebery were 21 hours and 5 minutes and my total solo hours 7 hours and 10 minutes. I was keen to continue my flying when I saved more money.

CHAPTER 2

REGULAR ARMY

I entered the Regular Army on the 24th July 1967 at an enlistment ceremony in St Kilda Road, Melbourne. Like other recruits, I took the Oath promising to defend the Constitution of Australia.

My army career started like everyone else's: the trial of training, the shaping of a soldier and the selection of postings. The training was fast and furious, the days long and exhausting at Kapooka Army Recruit Training Centre, situated outside Wagga Wagga New South Wales. I found the CMF training I'd undertaken as a teenager extremely valuable. In many ways, it helped me cope with the effort expected of me, and I was glad to have it under my belt. Physical training was exhausting, the hills punishing, and the place pushed me to my absolute limits. Kapooka had a reputation for toughness. Our only reprieve was on Sundays or when we had lectures, however if we fell asleep during lectures we had to stand for the rest of them as punishment.

Everything had to be perfect and completed on time. If anyone let the platoon down by failing the inspection, either of their gear or themselves, the whole platoon would be penalised.

Unofficially, we had our own in-house punishments – the platoon becoming judge, jury and executioner as we took our own disciplinary action. One rookie we'd nicknamed 'Sad Sack' let the platoon down countless times. He was scrubbed with icy water and a coarse bristle brush by several platoon members for not keeping sufficiently high cleanliness standards. Another rookie member considered a slacker was dealt with by having laxatives slipped into his Milo drink, tied to his bed and put outside on the parade ground one cold evening. He was in a fair state when he was finally retrieved the next morning. Both rookies' habits improved dramatically after their treatment. It was a hard lesson learned with harsh punishment, but it reflected the Army culture of the day with even the instructors encouraging and turning a blind eye to the bastardisation and bullying within the platoon.

We embarked on countless runs and forced marches wearing full kit along dusty dirt roads. It made no difference whether it was cold or raining. It certainly improved our fitness as well as encouraged us to work as a team. In retrospect, the runs and marches were essential, not only in improving our physical fitness, but in building the mental toughness to enable us to deal with conditions under duress. This significantly enhanced our chances of survival.

Before graduation I had to complete a 15-kilometre run without gear, followed by, the hardest by far, a 32-kilometre (20 miles) forced march with full gear which included webbing, bum-pack, belt, ammunition pouches, water-bottles, SLR, and taking turns in carrying the M60 machine gun. We were required to complete the march within a specified time. We were dropped off in the early morning at 0600 hours on a quiet country road about 32 kilometres from Kapooka and we started our march in dense fog. The air was still and cold. My frozen fingers wrapped round my SLR as low cloud threatened to engulf us. The first two or three kilometres went well as everyone managed to stay in formation, but as we progressed some rookies fell behind.

The day soon heated up and by midday, the sun was directly overhead. The heat burned into us and, with no breeze to provide relief, we struggled with the rising temperature and dehydration. To make matters worse, my feet slid around in my new boots and started chafing. I tried tightening the laces, but it did not help, and I soon developed blisters. For kilometres I experienced the agony of blisters breaking and redeveloping as I jogged along in full kit, every step forcing my face into a grimace of pain and determination. The platoon Lieutenant could see me struggling and asked if I wanted to quit. “No bloody way, Sir,” I gasped out, gritting my teeth. “I’m not letting this beat me, Sir.”

Half a dozen blokes from our platoon had already dropped out through heat exhaustion, aching feet and blisters, but I was determined not to be one of them. For the remaining kilometres I drew on every ounce of self-determination to rise above the heat and conquer the torture of my feet until, with enormous relief, I saw the main gates of Kapooka Army Barracks.

In my room I sat on the edge of my bed with my feet swollen and throbbing. My whole body screamed in agony as I tried to take off my boots. Two of my roommates, Whitey and Burgess, helped me to remove them and to our amazement, my socks and boots were soaked with blood, my feet a mass of weeping blisters. When I fronted the Army doctor at the Regimental Aid Post (RAP), he even raised his eyebrows as he applied antiseptic lotion and put me on light duties for five days during which time I hobbled around in thongs.

At the end of October 1967, 44 rookies including me graduated as soldiers. I ranked thirteenth in the platoon, felt a real sense of achievement and elected to join the Royal Australian Corps of Signals as my first choice.

The School of Signals was located at Balcombe on the Mornington Peninsula south of Melbourne. I wasn't due to start my Signal course until the beginning of 1968, so I was put into a Holding Troop where I was assigned various duties. For the next two months I was kept busy with duties such as shovelling dirt at an open dirt quarry into the tipper of a tip-truck, a kitchen hand known as a 'dixie-basher" in the Officers Mess, a steward in the Sergeants' Mess and finally a Batman for the Regimental Sergeant Major (RSM). The School of Sigs RSM was so impressed with me, he offered me the job full time with rank of Lance Corporal, but I felt it was boring and I wanted to achieve and learn more than being a Batman.

While working in the Sergeants' Mess as a steward, I again witnessed the ugly side of Army culture in bastardisation and bullying. The cook in the Mess had been demoted from Sergeant to Corporal, and was a bitter man who snarled out orders to me continuously. He had a grudge against this one Warrant Officer who had complained about the meals he was served previously. One evening I returned to the kitchen with the Warrant Officer's order for steak, mashed potato, mixed vegies and gravy. As the meal was prepared, I was shocked when the cook, who had a heavy cold, scraped his throat and spat out some yellow muck into the potato and covered it with more mashed potato. I stood beside him shocked and speechless. The cook instructed me, "Okay, you can serve him this meal now and I hope he bloody well enjoys it."

"But Corporal, this isn't right, you must be joking," I said.

"Shut up. Do your job or I will charge you and get the bloody order out," he shouted back at me. I went out to the dining room, and nervously placed the meal before the Warrant Officer then returned to the kitchen where the cook watched through a small servery window laughing his head off.

A few days after the incident the Warrant Officer came down with a bad case of the flu. It played heavily on my mind and I wondered what life in the Army was about.

The weeks passed quickly, and on Friday 15 December I headed back to Queensland on leave. It was just as well I'd started my leave when I did as two days later the Prime Minister, Harold Holt, disappeared while swimming in rough surf near Portsea. All the signallers and apprentices at Balcombe had their leave cancelled to search for our political leader. On 12 January 1968 my leave finally came to an end and it was time to head back to Melbourne by train. At Brisbane railway station I met another soldier who offered me a ride in his car to Melbourne. I foolishly accepted thinking the trip would be much quicker than the train. It was around 8.00pm when we finally began our journey, travelling through the night on the Pacific Highway at a breakneck speed and I was soon regretting my decision. He refused to slow down and just outside Grafton at around 6.00am in heavy rain our journey ended abruptly when our car veered across on the wrong side of the road hitting another oncoming car. I tried to brace myself by grabbing the back of the seat with my right hand as there were no seatbelts in those days. All I remember or heard was a ghastly crunch of metal. When I came to, I found myself sitting in a ditch by the side of the road with a large gash to my head and cheek, my left eye badly bruised and swollen. I must have been injured when my head hit the windscreen but thankfully no-one was seriously injured, just cuts and bruises. We were very fortunate as our car was still upright while the other car, containing a family of four was on its side. If the other car had not slowed down on the wet road to avoid a head-on collision, we probably wouldn't have been so lucky. Within a short time, the police, ambulance and tow trucks arrived. After being examined by the ambulance officers and questioned by the police, I grabbed a lift into Grafton, caught a bus to Sydney and then a train to Melbourne. I was still in shock and vomited several times on my way south. On my arrival at Balcombe, I was examined by a doctor and diagnosed with concussion and shock. I was given some tablets and a week off to recuperate.

Once again, I look back on my life and say, "Yes, that definitely is a PTSD symptom from a stressful event". To this day I still feel uncomfortable sitting in the front passenger seat, preferring the back seat.

The signals course commenced in late January. Soon I was immersed in learning to type telegraphic keyboards, set up telegraphic/radio equipment, operate different radio sets, understand radio and communications centre procedures and read telegraphic tapes. I enjoyed the intense four-month course immensely and in June 1968 I was posted to 139 Signal Squadron based at Enoggera in Brisbane, Queensland.

To my surprise, I learned that my twin brother Don and a close friend had enlisted in the Army. After Basic Training at Kapooka, he was selected for the Medical Corps with training conducted at Healesville in Victoria. It was an unexpected turn of events and this obviously caused our Mum to worry more with both her twin sons in the Army.

In August 1968 I was selected to attend a six-week cipher course back at Balcombe where I would learn to code and decode messages and use cipher machines. The course was held in an old wooden building in a small compound, surrounded by a high barbed-wire fence. The security was strict, and we were not permitted to take anything into the compound including bags, notebooks or pens. When we left for the day, the instructors checked our pockets to make sure we were abiding by the rules.

My cipher course concluded, and I attended a break-up party at the Mount Martha pub with four of our instructors and 11 other graduates. Sadly, this night I will remember the rest of my life. I was sexually assaulted by one of the instructors, a Staff-Sergeant who had spiked one of my drinks. When I complained I felt ill and dizzy he volunteered to take me back to Balcombe. "Come on soldier, I'll take you home. Reckon you've had enough," I vaguely remember him saying. He helped me to his car, and I must have passed out soon afterwards. When I came to my senses, I was horrified to find the Staff-Sergeant had unzipped my trousers and had his hand inside my shorts. It didn't take long for me to put two and two together and realised that he had spiked my drink.

"Sick bastard!' I yelled, shoving him aside. 'Get away from me, you sick cunt."

"If you report this, it'll be your word against mine," he said smugly. "And I'll make sure you never last in the Army."

He obviously hadn't expected me to wake up so soon. Then it dawned on me. The bloke had clearly done this before. I scrambled out of his car into the dimly lit Balcombe Army Signallers' car park. I felt sick and embarrassed, shocked by the whole incident. What the hell had he put in my drink? What effect would it have on me? I couldn't answer either question as I staggered away from his car, still feeling weak and blurry.

I was disgusted and angry, shaken and embarrassed. While I knew the Staff-Sergeant was a sick bastard, I was too embarrassed to say or do anything. I certainly didn't want to share my experience with anyone, nor did I want people to assume I'd played any willing part. The Army was important to me, and I didn't want to jeopardise my chances for promotion. Instead, I kept my mouth shut, told myself that his days were numbered and tried to put the whole business behind me. Chaotic thoughts swam through my mind. While I knew I should report the incident, the likely outcome was not encouraging.

That sexual assault affected me for the rest of my life. I question myself, "Why me?" Did I do something to encourage him? Could I have avoided it by coming across differently? Did I have a weak character? Was I at fault? All these questions are still with me to this day. I became angrier as

> *I got older. I could not talk about it to anyone. It affected my relationships with females. I lost all self-confidence within myself when going out socially meeting females. I felt worthless with low self-esteem and when I did get into a permanent relationship, I had periods of emotional numbness, no feelings. The biggest issue for me was feeling dirty after having sex. This reaction has never left me. It seemed to me I have been marked for life. I have flashbacks of the assault to this day especially when I view other victims' sexual assaults stories on television.*

On my return to 139 Signal Squadron my posting to Vietnam was confirmed for January 1969. I was only back at the Squadron for four weeks before going to Canungra to complete a four-week Battle Efficiency Course. Located some 70 kilometres south-west of Brisbane in the Gold Coast hinterland, the Jungle Training Centre was designed to replicate Vietnam. The conditions were physically tough, and we trained in the hot and humid Queensland summer.

We completed training in patrolling, map-reading and navigation in the steep, densely forested hills, learnt ambush and booby-trap techniques and fought mock battles at close range. A traditional Vietnamese village constructed of sticks and flimsy scraps of tin hedged with bamboo added an air of authenticity.

While our instructors lived in comfortable brick buildings, we lived in tents like the soldiers at Nui Dat. We had to run everywhere: to the mess, to the shithouse and to lectures. Every day was gruelling, filled with combat skills training, and obstacle courses in which we scrambled through barbed wire in full kit.

Explosions went off during mock battles, and we thrust our bayonets into sandbags. We had endless marches up 'Heartbreak Hill' and spent time on the rifle range.

The kilometre-long 'confidence course' tested us physically and mentally as instructors bombarded us with smoke grenades and we crawled under and over dozens of obstacles in full kit. There were tunnels to scramble through, barbed wire to negotiate, ropes to climb and at the end, a two-metre drop into a stinking soup of mud and slime populated with rotting kangaroo carcasses and urine. It was called 'the bear pit'.

Our training was fast coming to an end, but we faced one final operational test. That would be conducted over a period of a week in the Wiangaree State Forest in a semi-tropical forest known to the diggers as 'The Lost World'. To enter 'The Lost World' you had to descend around 200 metres to reach the bottom. The place was lost alright, kilometres of steep, forested, rugged country, deep valleys with thick jungle vines and lantana growing in impenetrable thickets. It rained the entire time we were stationed there, and we became accustomed to wearing wet clothes and dealing with leeches, ticks and mosquitoes. Most of us felt cold and miserable most of the time. The aim of the exercise was to learn to move and survive in the jungle, remain undetected and attack the 'enemy' (aka the training instructors from Canungra) when they least expected it.

Finally, our ordeal came to end, and I stepped out of the bush into the bright sunny world of Queensland. I felt exhausted and returned to my unit and soon afterwards was promoted to Lance Corporal. I was surprised and proud of my accomplishment in such a short time.

We got news my twin, Don, a member of the Medical Corps, was going to be posted to Vietnam in early 1969. Devastated to learn that both her twin sons were going to Vietnam at the same time, Mum approached the local Member of Parliament (MP). To everyone's surprise, the MP discovered some legislation which prohibited members of the same family serving concurrently in a war zone. The law had been introduced shortly after the sinking of the HMAS *Voyager* in 1964 in which several members of the same family had lost their lives. The MP brought the precedent to the attention of the Australian government which ordered a review of our posting. Don, as the older twin by seven minutes was expected to go to Vietnam. Instead, he went to Townsville while my posting to Vietnam remained. I suppose we'll never know how that decision was made. Don was visibly disappointed but held no grudges.

I began my pre-embarkation leave in mid-December with a mixture of excitement at being posted overseas on an adventure somewhere exotic in a tropical, undeveloped third world country while also fulfilling my duty to my country. During my two weeks of leave I had to reassure Mum constantly that I would be ok and not to worry but I knew deep down it wasn't working.

On the afternoon of 1st January 1969, I emotionally said goodbye to my Mum, twin brother, Don and friends and caught an overnight train to Sydney for our preparation for deployment to Vietnam at the Ingleburn Army Camp. At the camp, we sat through lectures on Vietnamese language and culture, had our final medical checks, inoculations, wrote our wills and were issued with our 'dog tags' which would stay with us from then on.

CHAPTER 3

TO VIETNAM

On Monday 6th January 1969 at 10.45pm I boarded the Qantas Boeing 707 with adrenalin and excitement coursing through my body for the 14-hour flight to Vietnam including brief stops at Darwin and Singapore.

After we boarded, we were given a white cardboard box containing an assortment of cut sandwiches, an apple and an orange. I sat next to my two rookie Kapooka training mates in Richard Burgess and Bill Scott. It was a high-spirited flight to Darwin. None of us got any sleep. My brain was too active as I thought of home and what Vietnam might be like. We arrived in Darwin in light rain and steamy hot conditions and waited in the empty airport terminal for an hour, before the plane departed for Singapore at 3.00 am.

Three hours later, we touched down in Singapore where we were instructed to change our Army shirts to white civilian shirts to appease the Singaporean officials. The tropical heat hit me like a furnace. Some officials directed us to a restricted area isolated from other passengers where for the next few hours, we played cards, read books or in my case caught up with some sleep on an uncomfortable wooden bench. I was awoken by an Australian Army Officer, "Morgan, you haven't had the right injections. You can either stay in Singapore or have a smallpox needle right now." I did not have much choice so I chose the latter, deducing that some medic at Ingleburn must have omitted to record it on my medical card. Three and a half hours later, I felt very inoculated with my double dose of smallpox vaccination as we left Singapore and two hours later, circled over Saigon.

My knuckles whitened around the arm of the seat as we made a steep descent to Tan Son Nhut airport Saigon, where it was hot and humid. As I waited at the terminal for my flight to Nui Dat with my uniform shirt crinkled with sweat, I viewed local Vietnamese people for the first time wearing conical straw hats and what looked like black silk pyjamas. I also could smell something like rotting vegetation and an occasional whiff of aviation fuel as a constant trail of aircraft landed and took off every few minutes.

After waiting about two hours at the terminal, I clambered up the rear-opening doors of the Hercules aircraft for the 20-minute flight to Nui Dat, the Australian Task Force base in Phuoc Tuy Province, 60 kilometres south-east of Saigon. We sat in a line along the fuselage on webbing slings with our gear stacked in the middle. It was like being in the belly of a huge noisy beast as everything creaked and shuddered when we hit pockets of hot turbulent air. Thankfully our flight was only short as at one stage I thought my eardrums would burst. We touched down at

Luscombe airfield strip at Nui Dat in the late afternoon.

Nui Dat meant 'small hill' in Vietnamese, was known to Australian servicemen as 'The Dat', and was the base camp for the Australian forces in Vietnam. It was camouflaged with scrubby growth and abandoned rubber plantations grown straggly and unkempt. The green-clad hill rose 60 metres above the surrounding terrain and provided an excellent view of the VC stronghold to the north-west.

The Vietnam War was a guerrilla war fought by the Viet Cong (VC) in the dense jungles of South-East Asia. It was a war without a front line. Scattered throughout Vietnam, the VC pursued strategies that consisted primarily of surprise attacks, ambushes, the use of booby traps and sabotage. The VC also used an extensive network of underground tunnels that enabled them to make surprise attacks and simply vanish back into the jungle.

My Vietnam experience had begun with 365 days and a wakey to go before I could return home to Australia. Thankfully when I arrived it wasn't monsoon season, and the base was dry and dusty and criss-crossed with red earthen roads.

I was allocated a bed in the tent city of our unit in the rubber plantation close to the helicopter pad. My tent was at the end of a row of trees which provided me a rare piece of shade. Tents were 2.5 metres apart and 4.5 metres square and neatly lined up in immaculate Army style. They were sandbagged to waist height which provided a blast wall in case of attack and each had a small pit hole or bunker outside the front flap.

All the tents contained four steel beds, a table and four chairs, four lockers, with the floor made of slatted wooden pallets while a single globe dangled from the central pole. My bed was in the far-right corner of the tent facing Kanga Pad. All the tents were connected to the others by duckboards made from disused wooden pallets.

Just by our tent lines was the canteen and theatre. An unpretentious building, the mess and kitchen consisted of an open shed with a tin roof where we had our meals while the theatre was an open-sided large tent.

Nearby was our Communications Centre (ComCen) and our admin building housed in huge steel sheds and protected by blast walls. Across the road from the ComCen was the 1st Australian Task Force (1 ATF) headquarters and the 83rd American heavy artillery battery.

I was shocked when I saw the shower and toilet block sheds. Four concrete dunnies with metal lids were raised on a rough slab of concrete. The dunnies sat side by side with no privacy partitions and the building was strewn with newspapers and magazines. I walked to the dunny at the far end and opened the lid. A powerful stench hit me as a swarm of flies erupted like a bomber squadron in full flight, and I peered down into the biggest shit hole I'd ever seen in my life.

In the shower block shed, I discovered four canvas bags hanging from the ceiling each with a shower nozzle at the base. They were connected by a pulley system to the tin roof trusses with a rope tied to the wall. It was a communal shower, all in together. For a shower you had to fill up a jerry can from a water tank trailer nearby and carry the container into the shower block, fill the canvas bag, pull the full bag up by a rope before turning on the nozzle below the bag.

We took a leak at the open communal urine pit known as a pissaphone. Pissaphones were located throughout the Nui Dat area. Some were in the open, situated near pathways or heavy traffic areas with no privacy. Others had some semblance of privacy with iron or tin sheeting or hessian. Ours was located near our shithouse or pit dunny. It had a tin sheet fence for privacy with a small gap for entry. It was constructed from a piece of water pipe with a funnel built into the pit hole itself surrounded by sand, gravel and rocks. The pit had a strange oily solution around the top of the hole.

Over the next few months, my embarrassment at all the shared toilet and washing facilities gradually faded, although I knew I would always have to take my chances with the 'shit flies' that lived and thrived in the dunny pit holes.

Within minutes of arriving at our tent lines, I became aware of the constant noise ... bucka, bucka, bucka ... as choppers landed and departed, booming sharp sounds from the US 83rd Artillery guns nearby or the tinny sound of transistor radios blaring from tents. I couldn't imagine I'd ever get used to the racket.

My first day in Vietnam ended. I felt buggered, clambering into my bed under a green mosquito net and on an uncommon firm mattress with a soft pillow. I felt homesick and uncomfortable from the overpowering heat. I couldn't sleep with the continuous booming sound from nearby artillery guns and was constantly on alert thinking every sound was the VC.

My second day began at around 0600 hours with the sun filtering through the rubber trees along with unremitting revving noise from choppers on Kanga Pad heading off on their various missions. After I gulped down my breakfast, I had to report to the Officer in Command of the ComCen, Warrant Officer Jock Bannigan. A Scotsman, Jock informed me that I would be going out forward to Fire Support Base (FSB) 'Julia' on Operation Goodwood in a few days. This came as a shock as I expected to stay and work at the ComCen.

After showing me through the ComCen, Jock then drove me around Nui Dat, a trip of around five kilometres. There was a lot to see, the place was full of activity. We visited the aerial farm with all the communication antennas, a small water dam, the PX building, the Salvation Army recreation building and the Regimental Aid Post (RAP). I began to get a feel for the place. It was huge, with a fortified perimeter of barbed wire and a five-kilometre defoliated zone. Men in jungle greens were everywhere and there were dozens of rows of tents among the straggly rubber trees.

On my return I went to the Q store, where I was issued with four sets of new jungle greens, an SLR (Self Loading Rifle) with ammunition, and some anti-malaria pills.

In mid-afternoon I accompanied other new members of 104 Sig Sqn to the Nui Dat rifle range to sight and range in our weapons.

The SLR was standard issue as a personal weapon in Vietnam. It was a reliable, hard-hitting, gas operated and magazine-fed semi-automatic rifle with an effective battle range of 300 metres. With a full 20-round magazine, it weighed 4.96 kilograms and had a practical rate of fire of 20 rounds per minute.

Having perfected our firing, we lined up to try our hand at the M60. This was an American general-purpose machine-gun with a bipod and an effective range of 500 metres or, with tripod,

1100 metres. The M60 was gas operated, air-cooled and belt-fed and had a quick-change barrel that prevented overheating during sustained firing. The M60 was the infantry section's main firepower in Vietnam and weighed 10.5 kilograms with a bipod and an extra 6.8 kilograms with a tripod.

The rifle range sergeant gave us some instruction on its use, and we stood in line waiting for our turn. I was behind Bruce Meakins, a mate from Enoggera and a member of 139 Signal Squadron. He and I had been on the same flight from Sydney. Bruce got into position took up the M60 and began firing, but the gun jammed.

'Bloody gun won't fire,' he yelled to the rifle range sergeant.

'Cock the weapon again, mate,' the Sergeant shouted.

Bruce cocked the M60 again, but with no success. When he tried to fire again, there was an explosion. Instinctively, I leapt away while Bruce screamed in pain and rolled around on the ground holding his bloodied and blackened face. It was like a bad dream, and we all yelled for what seemed like forever, but it was probably only a few seconds. Bruce calmed down, and I knelt beside him noticing that he had shrapnel wounds and burns to his face around his eyes. There was a lot of blood dripping from his face and two metal chunks protruded from his left eye. For an instant I thought he was going to die. We carried him to a Land Rover and the driver sped off to the Nui Dat RAP.

To our relief, I heard later that evening that Bruce was in a satisfactory condition and would stay in hospital for the next couple of weeks while his wounds healed. The accident had been caused by two rounds catching in the breech.

That night I couldn't sleep as my mind kept turning over the events of Bruce's accident. Images of him rolling around on the ground with his burnt and bloodied face, screaming in agony flooded my mind while I tossed and turned in my anxiety over the incident.

> ***This turned out to be my first horrific trauma or stressful incident in Vietnam that could have triggered my PTSD symptoms. Some incidents were more severe than others but they have all affected me in some ways with overwhelming feelings and emotions in depression, anxiety and anger spells.***

For the next couple of days, I worked in the ComCen from 0800 hours to 1700 hours. Our signals squadron supplied all the communication for the Task Force, including at the individual unit level. At least the ComCen was air-conditioned, and I could escape the stifling heat from outside. The centre ran 24/7 with eight soldiers on shift each day where Operators sent and received messages from Australia, Vung Tau and Saigon via teletype equipment. These machines produced a paper tape where each letter and symbol were represented by a pattern of holes and spaces across the tape called Murray code. Operators also encoded and decoded messages by Cypher equipment ensuring the enemy couldn't read the messages.

CHAPTER 4

FIRE SUPPORT BASE JULIA ON OPERATION GOODWOOD

I woke early on 11 January, keen to get ready for the convoy trip to a fire support base where I would be closer to the action. These bases were usually temporary firing bases carved out of the jungle and set up with an artillery battery, mortars and armour. They allowed a rapid and flexible response and greater coverage of operations beyond the immediate vicinity of the main Task Force base at Nui Dat. A fire support base sometimes remained in place for months and provided essential support to infantry field units and operations in remote areas.

They were named after officers' wives or girlfriends.

I loaded my pack and rifle onto the truck, and precisely at 0800 hours we rolled out of the main gates of Nui Dat. We passed the massive stone pillars at the entrance known as the 'Pearly Gates' as tanks and armoured vehicles led our convoy of trucks and Land Rovers laden with battle gear and personnel. Wearing basic webbing and holding our rifles with a few magazines of ammunition, we rumbled along on the right side of the road.

It was my first time beyond the perimeter wire, and I wasn't sure what to expect. I clutched my rifle as we passed through villages and hamlets. The locals watched as we passed on roads congested with vehicles. Trucks belched smoke, motor scooters, mainly Lambrettas, drove around like maniacal dodgems and buses were overloaded with passengers, baggage, wire cages crammed with squawking chooks and sacks of rice stacked precariously on the roofs. It was a scene of apparent confusion.

Villages and people flashed past in the dust as I saw chickens run and scratch in the dirt while peasants worked in paddy fields. All of them looked dilapidated and poor, lots of them wearing floppy black pyjamas and conical straw hats. The convoy rattled past several tiny single-storey houses made of mud, leaves and twigs. We saw ramshackle buildings fashioned from a combination of wood and rusty iron and occasionally we passed an elaborate house. The air was pungent with a strange fishy smell along with the ever-present stench of rotting vegetation.

A few kilometres further on we came to an abrupt halt. Part of the road, including a bridge, had been blown up by the VC. Fearing an ambush, we leapt off the trucks and I jumped into a ditch that dropped down steeply next to a paddy field.

For the next couple of hours, I remained crouching in the ditch with a few other soldiers on guard as infantry and armoured vehicles conducted a search and clearance patrol in the vicinity of the bridge while engineers looked for any disturbance on the road for mines or booby traps.

I clutched my rifle as the brutal reality of war enveloped me. This was my fifth day in Vietnam and my first time seeing the results of enemy destruction. Perspiring, I had mixed feelings and thought, "What on earth am I doing here in this stinking place?"

While in the ditch I noticed something shiny in the dirt by my boots. I discovered a silver aluminium Christian insignia ring with a crucifix on top and ten small fixed nodes around the ring which I assumed related to the Biblical Ten Commandments. In deep thought as I turned the ring over in my hand, I wondered who might have owned it and how this ring ended up in this insignificant ditch with me. Was it a sign of good luck? I placed it in my shirt pocket and decided it would be my good luck charm for rest of my tour.

> ***I eventually placed the ring next to my dog tags on a green nylon cord around my neck. A lot of soldiers had good luck charms to keep them safe, grounded and bring hope of returning home safely. I still have this Christian insignia ring with me to this day.***

After hours in the ditch, we received the all-clear and the engineers had constructed a temporary bridge. With no further delays we reached FSB Julia in mid-afternoon. It sat a few kilometres off the main highway between Nui Dat and Bien Hoa Province in a roughly levelled jungle clearing. We were allocated different areas to build sandbag protection, set up gun pits in our defensive area and construct our own personal pit holes. Julia was already well established with heavy equipment dropped in by Chinook helicopters. Bulldozers continued to clear the jungle scrub outside a heavily protected barbed-wire perimeter entanglement dotted with Claymore mines. We were relieved to see that our pit holes had already been dug, 1.5 metres deep by 1 metre wide, although we still had to fill sandbags to provide overhead protection.

After completing the overhead protection, I crawled down in a small gap at one end of my allocated pit hole to place my mattress and sleeping bag down the hole.

I had gone from a comfortable bed in Australia, to now sleeping in a hole in the ground like an animal.

Once we had our personal living arrangements sorted, we set up the signal centre. The communication equipment was already in place inside the Armoured Command Vehicle (ACV) where we would be working. All we had to do was erect a tent connected to the ACV, fill more sandbags and place them on top of the ACV for added protection. It was hot, sweaty work and physically demanding.

After completing the work, we headed over to the Task Force mobile field kitchen for some tucker where bugs, flies and swirling dust enveloped me.

Showers and toilets at the FSB were like at Nui Dat except that they were in the open with only a flimsy canopy fence for privacy. For showers we were only permitted half a canvas bag of water which lasted barely 30 seconds, but I guess it was better than nothing.

On my first night at FSB Julia, I had gun pit duty. This entailed working for two hours from 2200 hours before taking a break for four hours, and then being back on again from 0400 hours for another two hours. An M60 machine-gun on a tripod was set up in the pit and there was a remote trigger for the Claymore mines that were buried around the perimeter. Around the outside of the barbed wire entanglement that formed the perimeter fence were early warning devices known as trip flares. I was edgy and felt incredibly alone, despite having another bloke on duty beside me.

I sat in the gun pit in the blackness, tense and alert, not knowing what to expect. In the silence of the night I heard B-52s bombing in the distance and saw tracer bullets from helicopter gunships rip through the night skies. The hours passed slowly.

We heard strange noises, crackling and ripping sounds as if the whole jungle was on the move. After 2400 hours with my nerves on edge, I returned to my pit hole hoping to grab some sleep, but I struggled as it was stinking hot inside. At 0400 hours I was back on gun pit duty, like the first shift with noises from the jungle. By the time my shift ended, I was emotionally buggered.

> ***We never discovered what was making those noises. It was probably our imagination as we were in an anxious and hyper-aroused state of mind.***

I had the rest of the day off and returned to my pit hole hoping to grab some sleep. That was impossible, particularly with the barrage of nearby artillery firing, choppers flying in and out, plus the heat, dust, the bugs and flies.

Sleep deprived, the nights at Julia were perpetually noisy. The American artillery batteries fired their big howitzer guns a few hundred metres away, occasionally firing overhead to support the infantry battalions on operations and distant red and green tracer bullets from the helicopter gunships flicked through the night sky. It was like a massive out-of-control fireworks display.

Over the next couple of days, I quickly established a routine, starting work in the ACV at 1600 hours and finishing at 2400 hours in addition to daytime gun pit duties.

Working in the ACV was excellent as it was air-conditioned to keep our communication equipment cool. Each shift was eight hours, and I desperately wanted to stay there in the cool but as soon as my shift ended, I was out into the heat and dust again.

A couple of days later VC activity was reported in the area.

Late one afternoon I was on gun pit duty with my mate, Mal Jones (Jonesy) and another signaller. We watched as a Vietnamese peasant in black pyjamas picked up small pieces of wood and put them into a wooden cart pulled by a water buffalo.

The peasant was some distance away from the wire perimeter next to a cleared area recently graded by the Engineers. I didn't take much notice of the Vietnamese at first, thinking he was just a villager going about his local chores. However, as he moved closer to the wire and to where we sat in the gun pit, my interest increased sharply. My mates and I watched him for 30 minutes before Jonesy spoke.

"I reckon this bloke is a bloody Viet Cong, he's checking out the strength on our perimeter."

"Yea, Jonesy. You may be right," I said not entirely convinced. "He sure fits the bill in those bloody black pyjamas. Mind you they all wear them."

The peasant moved closer to the wire.

"I reckon we should fire a bloody warning shot over his bloody head, don't you? That should scare the bugger off," Jonesy piped up.

At this stage, I was getting nervous, so without further hesitation, I took Jonesy's advice and fired a few rounds from the M60 machine-gun into the foliage. I'd never seen anyone move as fast. The suspected VC stumbled in his attempt to get away from the perimeter area, fell in a hole and dropped half his pile of wood. As he scrambled out, he tried desperately to hang onto his out-of-control buffalo. We never confirmed if he was a VC.

For the next few days the weather continued hot and humid. I didn't know how anyone could enjoy living in these conditions with the heat and the mugginess day and night. The place was the absolute pits with the dust dreadful. Living in the dirt, always made many of us secretly wish we'd never come to Vietnam. When you sweated, you became aware of the dirt that constantly coated your body. You could never get rid of it.

Over the past few days, my eyes had become excessively bloodshot, my eyelids red and crusty with a yellow discharge. I wasn't sure whether it was the sun, the dust or the heat, or some combination of all three, but I knew I had an infection. I visited the RAP where the medic diagnosed a severe case of conjunctivitis brought on by dust and dirt and gave me some antibiotic ointment to apply at night.

My discomfort was nothing compared to other soldiers who were suffering heat rashes and constantly itching and scratching themselves, poor buggers. Prickly heat and skin conditions like crotch rot around your genitals were a real health concern. Thank God I didn't have that.

Filling sandbags, digging pit holes, or going out on clearing patrols exacerbated skin conditions. Some of the blokes had developed eczema from the heat, and I heard of one soldier who had to be medevaced out (evacuated) due to the severity of his condition.

Every night I developed my own routine to prevent such conditions by using unlimited amounts of Army issue talcum powder in and around my armpits, genitals and feet. I'd repeat the procedure again in the morning.

> ***The practice was something I maintained the whole time I was in Vietnam in the hope it would prevent crotch rot or something equally distasteful.***

A week later, I began the 0800 hours to 1600 hours shift in the ACV, with the big American guns maintaining a barrage for days firing at a camp of 60 VC nearby. Dozens of VC had already been slaughtered, and we'd had a few casualties too, when an Armoured Personnel Carrier (APC) went over a mine killing a crew member and wounding a couple of soldiers.

After another lengthy exchange of fire, several wounded Aussie Infantry soldiers arrived at FSB Julia by chopper. A couple were subsequently air-lifted, their greens torn to shreds, filthy and spattered in blood. Five Australians had died in the action and were now zipped into body bags awaiting an incoming chopper. It was a rude awakening to the reality of war.

Two hours before midnight, just as I was settling down for the night, the VC attacked the perimeter fence. Night turned to daylight as flares were set off around the base and tracer bullets whizzed about wildly. I grabbed my rifle and peered out through the small opening of my pit hole. Loud cracking and booming noises radiated from the APC and the gun pits nearby. Tracer bullets darted overhead. My muscles tensed, hairs bristled on the back of my neck as I crouched and fidgeted with my rifle and readied for action. The battle lasted 20 minutes although it felt like an eternity. Then all went quiet as we remained on full alert. An hour and a half later, the attacks recommenced, each skirmish lasting around 20 minutes. Our Commanding Officer reckoned it was a small group of Viet Cong who had infiltrated the area as far as to our perimeter wiring and who were using small arms fire to pepper us before retreating. Thankfully, there were no casualties, but we were all buggered by the experience.

I spent another busy day in the ACV, as night approached. FSB Julia remained on a knife edge, with all of us anxious about what the darkness would bring. Sure enough, the VC attacked repeatedly over the next three nights. Each time the confrontations caused my nerves to be on edge, with fear especially, waiting to be attacked. Clearing patrols went out but failed to locate the VC.

At midnight on the third night, I finished my shift and headed to my pit hole. I was both physically and emotionally exhausted. Relieved I was not on gun pit duty, I soon dropped into a deep sleep. Like clockwork, the VC attacked two hours later with small arms fire and mortar shells fired directly into the base. I was instantly awake when there was a God-almighty explosion as a mortar landed just metres from my pit hole. My pit hole collapsed, dirt, gravel the whole works. My whole world was caving in on top of me. It felt as if tons of heavy dirt, sandbags, and rusty iron sheeting were crushing me. My ears were pierced with pain as my world turned black and I struggled to breathe. In a panic, I thrashed around in all directions. When I discovered my feet were free, I kicked wildly as the instinct to survive took over, and I thrust my body forward. By now, I had lost all sense of time and had no idea how long I'd been there. I moved to the right of the pit hole and pushed with all my might. I finally managed to heave and roll myself sideways before forcing myself up, propelled by an overwhelming fear that I would be buried alive. The sandbags, dirt, poles and iron sheets collapsed to the left as I pushed my way to freedom. Everything was happening in slow motion. Consumed with adrenalin, I grabbed my rifle and made a desperate dash for the gun pit ten metres away with red tracer bullets whizzing over my head. The place was chaotic as guns fired from all around.

"Morgan, you silly bastard," Signaller Brian O'Neill yelled as I jumped into the pit beside him. "What the fuck are you trying to do? Get your bloody head shot off? You crazy bastard!"

Covered in cuts and abrasions to my head and face, I sat shaking and dry retching in the gun pit hole with two other soldiers until the tracer bullets eventually stopped coming. After two hours in the gun pit, I realised the adrenalin rush had fuelled my escape from my pit hole and my flight through VC gunfire to the gun pit. I couldn't believe I was alive. Never for a moment had I contemplated how dangerous my run had been. Not only had I put myself in a position of danger I'd also put my fellow soldiers in a situation where they could have killed one of their own. When I'd jumped out of the pitch-black night into that gun pit, they had been fumbling for their knives ready to take out the enemy intruder. I'd escaped my nightmare only to become theirs.

Luck was the distance between life and death.

When dawn broke, I went to the first-aid tent for observation but was back on duty within a couple of hours. My first task was to rebuild my pit hole and strengthen it. My mind raced in all directions wondering what I was doing as thoughts of never being able to get down in a pit hole ever again flooded my brain. For the next few nights and days this was the case as, choosing to take my chances with the VC, I slept on a stretcher on top of my pit hole rather than the suffocating depths down in it. In hindsight, this was not a smart decision, but it was one that every nerve in my body told me was the best one for me.

My brain kept hammering that I should get down in my pit hole and not be a wimp. With sheer determination, I eventually made it down, but I was never comfortable again, always anxious when there were any explosions or gunfire. My sleep and dreams were always recapturing the moment of not being able to breathe, and the whole world falling in on top of me. My pit hole now felt like a grave.

> ***Though I didn't know it at the time, that night changed my life forever. After 50 years it continues to haunt me during my sleep, in the form of a violent nightmares along with other PTSD symptoms.***

The hot, sweaty days in the jungle at FSB Julia passed slowly. My eyes continued to give me trouble, brought on by the swirling dust churned up by the tanks that rolled through the camp.

A week later, the Americans dropped hundreds of brochures written in Vietnamese. Written in bold print across the top were the words 'Chieu Hoi' which translated as 'To surrender'. The aim was to persuade the VC to surrender with the promise they would be treated kindly. It didn't work as in late January the VC hit us again. While all contacts were relatively brief, the action with the enemy was enough to rattle our nerves.

Two weeks later, on an exceptionally dark night with just a sliver of a new moon. I was on gun pit duty from 2000 hours to 2200 hours when we heard weapons firing a short distance from the perimeter. Our Infantry platoon had ambushed the VC. Another soldier and I set off flares hoping to deter any further attacks on us.

By then, I'd been at FSB Julia for a month. It seemed like forever. Towards the end we had a couple of quieter days before another nine Aussies died with ten seriously wounded in the nearby jungle. I was constantly on edge, my mind filling with anxiety as I considered the terrifying consequences of an attack, knowing at any stage, that it could be me, wounded or in a body bag.

Four weeks and three days after arriving at FSB Julia, Operation Goodwood concluded. Relieved, I gathered and packed my gear, dumped dirt from sandbags into my pit hole, and dismantled tents and coiled lengths of barbed wire. It took us a couple of hours to load everything onto the trucks before we returned to Nui Dat by convoy.

CHAPTER 5

BACK TO NUI DAT

Sweaty and dirty, I was looking forward to some time off, but told I would be working immediately in the ComCen for the next week on night shift from 1730 hours to 0730 hours. It was a rotating roster with one week of night shifts, one week of day shifts and one week on gun pit and working party including a couple days off in that week. I was the shift leader and supervised seven signallers.

After a while, it all became mundane, boring and predictable but despite the heavy workload I felt grateful Nui Dat was quieter and safer than FSB Julia.

I looked forward to receiving mail from home as it lifted my spirits and helped me to carry on. I was not alone. Letters were important to all of us, a link to the outside world, reinforcing the vital fact that no-one had forgotten us.

Mum wrote to me every week and sent me four Melbourne Herald-Sun newspapers every month. I was devastated and angry when told the posties and wharfies had gone on strike back home, delaying mail, equipment and stores. All the soldiers in Vietnam were upset, so some of us decided to print on our letters 'whack a wharfie' or 'punch a postie' for retaliation to get the message across.

The week on Work Party duties we were allocated different duties, such as filling blast walls, garbage runs, water supply runs, general clean ups around our area, maintenance work, gun pit duties and riding shotgun on convoys etc.

If I was lucky to get a day off, I'd spend the entire day catching up on sleep, writing letters, visiting the PX canteen or perhaps going for a swim at the most popular place at Nui Dat, the 5 RAR pool. It was an exhausting regime.

For my nights off I'd visit our canteen boozer for a couple of beers (two cans a day was our ration but not while on operations), and then watched a movie in the open tent theatre next to the boozer. The highlight of the week for me was the Saturday night BBQ, mainly because it was the only meal I enjoyed all week. The rest of the meals were rubbish, particularly breakfast. The scrambled eggs tasted disgusting. Eggs in Vietnam were freshened with ether.

My deckchair became my faithful friend, accompanying me to the movies, the boozer, the squadron barbeque on Saturday nights, tent parties and concerts at Luscombe Bowl. At times, deckchairs made perfect weapons, particularly in boozer punch-ups. It was a common sight to see soldiers trudging along the duckboards early in the evening clutching their simple but valuable piece of property.

Luscombe Bowl was an amphitheatre known as the 'Dust Bowl' where we enjoyed concerts. During my time at Nui Dat, I went to several concerts featuring some great comedians and singers. It was the best entertainment and provided some respite from the ever-present dangers.

It was uncharacteristically quiet at Nui Dat but this changed on the 23rd February at 0315 hours, I was having a rare and beautiful sleep when the siren went off and all hell broke loose. Mortar and rocket fire were raining down on Nui Dat. My fellow tent mates Nev Roberts, and Boobla Hegarty and I dived out of bed, pulled on our greens, grabbed our rifles and a couple of additional magazines and darted into our pit hole.

"And which of you dirty bastards are pissing and chucking your beer cans in the bloody pit hole?" Nev said, surveying the collection of empty beer cans.

"Well, it's not me," I said.

Boobla was more direct. "Stop fucking whinging, Nev. We're bloody well under attack. We're lucky to have any protection over our heads. Anyway, it's probably you, you dirty bastard."

The three of us waited, the mental and physical strain evident in our faces while the stench of urine was overpowering. I had to agree with Boobla. A few stray beer cans were nothing compared to what was happening at ground level as explosions blasted around us and we heard the crack of gunfire as flares ignited and mortars erupted.

We remained in the pit hole for three and a half hours. When we emerged, we heard that the VC rocket and mortar fire had left craters at the entrance to Nui Dat, also the aerial farm with all the antennas had suffered some minor shrapnel damage.

Fortunately, there was no other major damage.

Next day, the 24th, WO Jock Bannigan (he was the local bookie) told me I would be going to Saigon later that day to collect some cipher gear. I caught a flight to Saigon. A Signal driver met me at Tan Son Nhut airport and took me to the Australian Signal Centre in downtown Saigon. The traffic had to be seen to be believed as hordes of bicycles, Honda motor scooters and dinky blue and yellow Renault taxis swarmed through the streets.

The traffic appeared to move as one, and I wondered how on earth we would get through.

"What's this?" I asked as I was handed a metal briefcase with a handcuff chain at the Signal Centre.

"What's it bloody well look like, Corporal? It's a handcuff with chain attached to a bloody case. It's a precaution in case some idiot tries to knock it off. Stops you from losing the whole bloody thing."

I slipped the chain around my wrist. The case felt solid and heavy.

"What's inside?" I asked.

The reply, "A small cipher machine, cipher key rings and a few cipher cocks."

I arrived back at Nui Dat in the evening to find Jock waiting and looking anxious.

"Good work, well done, Morgan." he said, unlocking the handcuff.

I never did find out what was in the metal case, but I had a few theories. I reckon it was more of a bookie run than a cipher run as it certainly made Jock happy.

That evening the warning siren at Nui Dat sounded and once again we had to retreat to our pit holes as incoming rockets whizzed through the air and exploded within the perimeter of Nui Dat. Despite the chaos, no-one died.

It was now 4th March 1969. I had been in Vietnam for eight weeks. It seemed like eight years. I was due to celebrate my 21st birthday but my 21st party treat was being in a work party, taking disused timber down to the dump, after which I had gun pit duty, a solemn 21st for me.

A few days later, I was ordered to go to another fire support base.

CHAPTER 6

FIRE SUPPORT BASE KERRY ON OPERATION FEDERAL

FSB Kerry was in Bien Hoa Province near Long Binh, the large American base. I left Nui Dat early morning on the 9th of March by Iroquois chopper, my first chopper flight in Vietnam. I was enveloped in the shuddering rhythm that every Vietnam soldier would instantly recognise. We flew low over paddy fields, broken jungle, river deltas, canals and rough terrain dotted with small villages and towns.

The trip to FSB Kerry took 35 minutes, reaching the jungle clearing 55 kilometres north of Nui Dat and 25 kilometres north-east of Saigon. The chopper clattered to a stop, the rotor blades whooshing as I stepped out in a world of dust.

The set-up was like at FSB Julia, working in the Armoured Command Vehicle (ACV), manning the gun pit and doing escort duty for convoy runs to the American base at Long Binh.

As soon as I arrived, I was informed that I was on a clearing patrol later that afternoon. In the meantime, I constructed my pit hole with my thoughts instantly flashing back to FSB Julia when the pit hole had collapsed on top of me. Emotionally I was still not over it – looking down into it was like looking into my empty grave.

At 1700 hours I reported with 11 others for my first clearing patrol wearing my 'giggle' hat (light cotton hat) and my green Army scarf.

For some reason, I'd missed out on a clearing patrol at FSB Julia. In addition to my rifle, I had a couple of water canteens, a ration pack, my basic webbing, a few magazines of ammo, a bayonet in a pouch and an entrenching tool. The entrenching tool was a fold-up shovel and pick combo.

We left the heavily barbed-wire perimeter fence and moved out 300 metres into the dense jungle to check the immediate area for VC activity. Adrenalin was rushing through my body. I felt anxious and tense and was sweating profusely as we trod slowly and silently through broken trees and jungle foliage. From time to time we stopped to listen, and I took the opportunity to mop sweat from my eyes and forehead with the Army scarf that dangled around my neck. For an hour and a half, I remained on full alert as we cleared half the sector of the base while another patrol cleared the other half. Neither patrol found any evidence of VC and we returned to the perimeter fence with nothing to report.

For the next couple of days, I was detailed to other clearing patrols, relieved each time we returned with nothing to report. Back at the fire support base, I continued doing shift work in the

ACV Signal Centre plus a couple of gun pit duties. I was getting used to life with interrupted sleep. Sleep was a luxury. Despite the noise of choppers and guns, and the flares that illuminated the jungle at night, I always tried to catch a couple of hours between duties.

After a week at FSB Kerry I got my first escort duty for a convoy doing a Q Run (stores supply) to fetch water, rations and laundered greens from the large American Air Force Base at Long Binh. Sitting next to a driver with my Self-Loading Rifle at the ready, we set off in a Land Rover towing a trailer. On our way we stopped at a Catholic Vietnamese orphanage to give little children chocolate bars, tinned food and biscuits from our unused ration packs. I glanced around at the dozens of little sad faces who had lost their parents through greed and war. Their little faces quickly turned to grins.

At Long Binh, we collected the stores, food packs, and mail and delivered a pile of dirty greens to the laundry. It took all afternoon. On our return to FSB Kerry we saw two road accidents but the convoy continued as we were not permitted to stop.

In mid-March the VC began their third offensive. From 15th to 23rd March they hit us hard with rocket, mortar and small arms fire every night. They also hit some of the surrounding towns and bases, including Xuan Loc, some eight kilometres away. The VC always attacked at night, forcing us to remain on constant alert. I was on gun pit duty with another signaller on 18th March when we set off flares, some Claymores and fired the M60 machine-gun into the jungle foliage on our perimeter sector. Though we never saw them, we knew the VC were out there somewhere. That feeling of being watched could make the hairs on your neck stand on end and have your nerves screaming with anticipation.

The Australian Rock 'N' Roll singer Normie Rowe and his mates were in the APC next to our gun pit hole. Like us they were firing directly into the jungle foliage from a high-calibre machine-gun mounted on top of their APC. Most skirmishes lasted ten to 15 minutes before all was quiet again. However, the big artillery guns boomed all night, and along with fire from the gun pits and APCs setting off occasional flares, our camp was lit up like a fairground.

I was buggered. The stress of being constantly on alert, coping with the constant barrage of guns firing as well as the endless hot and humid weather, was taking a toll on me. To make matters worse, it started to rain which made the following day even hotter and steamier.

Our Commanding Officer, Major Morel, was very good and understanding. He would give a couple of the troops a night off in Long Binh. It was my turn and I could barely contain my excitement. I left at noon by Q vehicle and stayed at the 53rd American Signal Battalion barracks. At Long Binh, a sprawling base with luxurious accommodation compared to Nui Dat, the Yanks had everything, including hot and cold water, proper showers and toilets, TV, movies, floor shows and a mess open 24 hours.

First stop for me was the local barber shop where a Vietnamese man gave me a stylish crew cut. I returned to the barracks where I had a hot shower for the first time since leaving Australia and flopped onto a soft, comfortable bed and went into a deep sleep.

I was awoken by an American soldier, "Eh, man, you want to get something to eat?" he asked in a friendly drawl.

"Thanks, mate," I said as I leapt from my bed and followed him to the air-conditioned mess. At the mess I enjoyed some excellent food and plenty of ice-cold water. The cooks offered a couple of choices, or you could serve yourself and eat as much as you liked. After a satisfying meal, I sloped off to watch a TV broadcast in an air-conditioned lounge with comfortable cushion-backed seats.

My newly acquired American friend then took me to the Air Force Club where we watched a floor show of South Vietnamese 'go-go' dancers and I chatted to a few other Americans. They were fascinated by my Aussie accent and quizzed me about life 'down under', several eager to visit on their next R&R (rest and recreation) leave.

I left at around 2230 hours. After a quick shower, I was in bed again enjoying a soft mattress and no artillery fire. At around 0200 hours there was a huge explosion. I was instantly awake and leapt out of bed. For a second I thought I was back at FSB Kerry or FSB Julia as my heart raced and I searched in the dark for my rifle.

"Don't worry, it's quite normal," the bloke in the next bed drawled as he switched on the lamp beside his bed. "Just incoming mortar fire from the VC. They attack the airfield and hangars, all the time, man."

I was exhausted and tried to sleep, but it was nigh on impossible with mortars exploding at close range. Fatigue must have eventually overcome me, and I managed to grab an hour or two sleep before the Q vehicle collected me at 1000 hours.

I arrived back at FSB Kerry and went straight back to my normal routine, working in the ACV, gun pit duties, clearing patrols and had the usual disturbed sleep. I momentarily wondered if going to Long Binh had all been a dream.

On the late afternoon the 21st March I took out a clearing patrol. On our return to the perimeter barbed wire I checked my rifle and pointed it to the sky, took the entire magazine off and cocked the weapon to ensure there were no bullets in the breech before firing. I'd developed the bad habit of resting the barrel of the rifle on my boot when I pulled the trigger. To my horror an explosion reverberated through my boot.

"Contact!" the clearing patrol yelled in unison as everyone dropped to the ground. 'Fuck, where did that come from?'

"It's okay," I yelled, standing in a cloud of dust, "it came from my weapon. I've had a fucking AD (accidental discharge)."

Another signal operator, John Bertini, was in front of me. John was shaking, his face bone white. "Fuck you, Morg, I've just shit myself. I thought you'd shot me."

"Sorry, John, I must've cocked it with the magazine still on. Unless it was a double feed or something wrong with my SLR?"

I repeated myself several times to convince myself what had happened as the patrol scrambled back to its feet. Everyone was visibly relieved that it wasn't the VC. I was embarrassed at my slackness and lack of concentration. I felt like digging a hole and jumping in. I apologised to John and the other clearing patrol members knowing I could have killed someone or shot my foot off. I was automatically charged and fronted Major Morel the next morning at 0900 hours.

After a brief discussion, the Major found me guilty and gave me a severe tongue lashing followed by a stern warning. I was more upset when my SLR was found to be in perfect working order. I had caused the accidental discharge by being careless and irresponsible and was fined $40.

The Task Force expected the VC to increase their offensive over the next few days. Rocket and mortar fire had already hit many towns and bases during the night including FSB Kerry. The usual VC tactic was to come in close to the base at night and fire a few rounds before retreating into the jungle. Two clearing patrols left at dawn and again just before sunset. One turned clockwise while the other went anti-clockwise.

I was on the dusk patrol that left late afternoon. We were returning to base when Signaller Kevin Eickenloff saw something moving in the broken jungle foliage. We all hit the ground. For several minutes we listened and watched for the slightest sound or movement as we lay motionless, hardly daring to breathe. It seemed like hours.

Given the all-clear, we set off again. Moments later, we observed more movement. We dropped to the ground again. For five minutes we tried not to breathe as we watched carefully for the smallest movement or sound. We scrambled back to line formation and heard more movement in the broken jungle. It turned out to be the other Australian Task Force patrol. They saw us at the same time we saw them. After a lot of yelling by forward scouts from both sides, it dawned on us that it was a near miss of friendly fire. The other patrol had failed to return to base the correct way. It could so easily have ended in disaster.

In late March the heavens opened, and it rained continuously for three hours without a break. I'd never seen anything like it before. It caused havoc at the fire support base. I slithered into my pit hole to get some protection, but after a while the rain seeped through the sandbags, small at first then finally poured in like a flowing creek. I had to move myself with my sleeping bag and gear and join others at the open tent mess. Some of us took our shirts off and enjoyed the pounding of the cool rain as the dust turned to red mud. After the deluge, everywhere I walked my boots were loaded with mud while the tanks, APCs and motor vehicles churned the soaked ground into a quagmire.

The afternoon and evening monsoonal rains continued unabated for the next couple of days. My pit hole was waterlogged so I reverted to sleeping on my stretcher on top of my pit hole. At least there was no contact with the VC. Perhaps the wet weather had dampened their spirits.

Ten days had passed since my last visit to the American base at Long Binh. It was my turn to go and it came at a perfect time as I was exhausted with hardly any sleep. Again, the Yanks treated me like a King. This time I had a good night's sleep with no VC firing and no interruptions.

When I returned to FSB Kerry the next morning, I was told we would be moving to FSB Jillian on Operation Overlander in a couple of days. Feeling a little refreshed, I was back to my normal routine of duties. I discovered my pit hole had dried out and I could enjoy a decent sleep. I was in a deep sleep when suddenly I was wide awake. Something was moving in my pit hole. I listened intently and it sounded like a scratching sound. I fumbled for my torch and observed a scorpion as big as my fist at the end of my pit hole. Without any further provocation, I leapt out and slept the remaining hours on my stretcher. At dawn I undertook an exhaustive search of my pit hole, moving sandbags top and bottom but to no avail.

On the 3rd April, once I finished work in the ACV at 0800 hours it was time to pack my gear before destroying my pit hole by cutting open the sandbags with my machete and emptying the dirt down the hole. Then I helped load the trucks with communication gear, tents, barbed wire and boxes of ammunition. Just over three hours later, we left FSB Kerry for the jungle to reclaim.

CHAPTER 7

FIRE SUPPORT BASE JILLIAN ON OPERATION OVERLANDER

The two-hour trip by convoy to FSB Jillian, north of Saigon in Bien Hoa Province was, thankfully, uneventful. We travelled south for 25 kilometres on Route Two and passed through the usual villages until we finally reached the hole in the jungle known as FSB Jillian. Surrounded by rubber plantations and devastated jungle, it wasn't as dusty as Kerry and was much cooler. We were immediately back into the hard slog of unloading gear and setting up the Signal Centre in an ACV. Some 17 contacts had been reported in the area the previous day, six VC had died and four had been wounded. With our adrenalin pumping, we were immediately on full alert as we worked fast and furiously to create protection for ourselves.

With nothing dug for our pit holes, long ammunition boxes and galvanised sheeting that resembled half-sized tanks were substitutes for our new home away from home. We arranged all the ammo boxes and tanks in a line before filling hundreds of sandbags with dirt and placing them on top for added protection. When we'd finished it looked like a line of dog kennels, and we dubbed it the 'doghouse'.

My new bed was in an ammo box with enough room to slide in and out, either head or feet first. I always felt overwhelmingly claustrophobic. Bigger blokes settled into the comfort of the half-tanks.

We secured the area and built gun pits and I started work in the ACV at 1730 hours, working through to midnight. By this time, I'd been awake and working for 25 hours straight.

The following day it was Good Friday, 4 April 1969. We were informed that the Minister for the Army was arriving later in the day. I was in the ACV most of the day as the infantry brought in a few VC from a nearby contact a few kilometres away. The VC were blindfolded, and one was wounded and lay groaning on a stretcher in dirty black pyjamas before being taken to the Intelligence Corps area for questioning.

Just after noon the chopper arrived with the Army Minister aboard. We watched as he stepped out into the dust and shook hands with a few high-ranking officers. With a major contact going on nearby, the chopper barely wound down before it took off again and headed to Saigon.

On Easter Saturday I was sent on a cipher run, my first cipher run to change codes on the radio sets at several fire support bases including Sally (5 RAR, 105 Field Battery), Wattle (9 RAR, 161 Field Battery), Xuan Loc and Tran Bom. At each fire support base, I had to change the sets (KY-38 Secure Voice System) with a key change plunger. The plunger was the size of a milk bottle and had a handle on top and an assortment of spikes set to the 'up' or 'down' position by the cipher operator. My job was to push the plunger into each radio keyhole to change the code of each set.

> ***Cipher runs entailed the Cipher Sergeant and Cipher Corporal changing the daily key settings of Australian radio sets at fire support bases and Logistic Support Detachments with American and South Vietnamese forces. We travelled either on trucks and Land-Rovers on the roads or by choppers and fixed wing aircraft to up to eight locations.***

I clambered aboard the two-seater Sioux helicopter nicknamed 'Possum' that looked like a glass bubble. I was briefed by the pilot on safety and emergency procedures and informed that my job was to survey the ground for any VC activity. For two hours we skimmed the jungle, rubber plantations, paddy fields and small villages. I saw numerous fire outbreaks from artillery fire and bombing raids and heard B-52 bombers droning in the distance.

The following day I completed another cipher run, this time to Nui Dat by Iroquois chopper to collect some cipher gear. The trip took 15 minutes each way. After collecting the cipher gear and on our way back to FSB Jillian we saw several explosions and contacts with the VC with the gunners having to yell above the noise of the chopper for us to hear.

FSB Jillian was like the other fire support bases. Flares lit the jungle at night and there were always a few close VC contacts.

An infantry patrol brought in two prisoners and I finally saw the enemy up close. Barefooted, their faces were filthy and their black pyjamas grubby. They looked younger than me. The Infantry passed them over to the Intelligence Corps at Task Force Headquarters next to our ACV Signal Centre where they were to be interrogated. Later that day, the two prisoners, blindfolded and their hands tied behind their backs, were escorted by two intelligence officers to a chopper and flown to Nui Dat.

In the second week of April there was a lot of contact with the VC in the area surrounding the fire support base with significant chopper activity in and out of the base, particularly when 9 RAR and 5 RAR found an enemy bunker three kilometres from Jillian. Two 9 RAR boys died and 13 were wounded while ten VC were killed. I was busy in the ACV Signal Centre sending out notices of casualties which reported how many soldiers had been killed or wounded, and details of the contact.

Four days later, we packed up the base, ripped open the sandbags and left the stinking jungle to return to Nui Dat.

CHAPTER 8

BACK TO NUI DAT, ON CIPHER RUNS AND DAILY ROUTINE

By now I'd been in Vietnam for 14 weeks, most of my time spent at fire support bases. Relieved to be back in the relative safety of 'the Dat', I soon discovered that there was no down time as I was a shift leader in the ComCen. With responsibility for managing the shift, I also checked that work was completed and solved problems as they arose.

For relaxation, in my spare time I recorded or taped music from other soldiers or from the American Forces Vietnam Network. The Network theme was 'The Beat Goes On', and they played some excellent music.

From 28 April to 6 May, I attended a Subject 'A' course for corporal rank. It was a full-time course and was attended by selected members from various corps units at Nui Dat. I was nominated by my squadron and felt glad that we were not being disadvantaged by missing promotion courses while on active service. The course consisted mostly of drills and weapons instruction and, at the conclusion, I'd be assessed on drill movements with arms on the parade ground.

Encouraged by the success of passing my Subject 'A' course presentation, I decided to attend a Subject 'C' course on military law for two hours each day from Monday to Friday. Gun pit duty, cipher runs, and shift work made it difficult for me to juggle course attendance and study, but I still planned to sit the exam which was held at 0930 hours on Saturday 17 May.

I was busy on cipher runs, as whenever the infantry on Operations needed to change settings on their new secure radio sets, I had to go out to different areas by chopper or road convoys. My job as a signaller was to secure the KY-38 radio sets every day and provide a secure net, making it impossible for the VC to listen in. It was a difficult time as there was a surge in VC attacks with mortars, and rockets hit towns like Dat Do and some of the bases I visited.

Towards the end of May, it started raining heavily. The deluge typically started in the early hours of the morning. With no proper drainage system around the ComCen, we used heavy industrial brooms to get rid of the water and mud that constantly flooded the centre. Despite our efforts, the place was soon a quagmire. We had no other option but to dig a deep drain on our next work party day.

Fortunately, our tents were okay. The main problems were humidity, mud and the local insect life. In the evening when we turned the lights on in our tents we would be swamped by a rush of flying ants and bugs.

Two days later, Major Morel granted six signallers including me two nights in Vung Tau at the Australian Peter Badcoe Club. It would be my first decent break in Vietnam, and I was looking forward to having three days off.

Major Morel called the six of us together and gave us a short lecture on the dangers of Vung Tau, particularly the brothels, prostitutes and the bars.

With the high rate of venereal disease (VD) among soldiers in Vietnam, the Major gave us a list of supposedly healthy bars, adding that there were no guarantees and to be careful. Rumours abounded including one story about an Australian digger who had got the worst case of VD, called 'The Blackjack'. I was told parts of his penis went gangrenous before he finally shot himself, also about prostitutes being Viet Cong agents and how they concealed razor blades inside their vaginas.

After lunch on the 21st May, six of us left the main gate in a convoy of trucks and Land Rovers. Vung Tau was 40 kilometres away, and we travelled at speed, passing through the town of Baria and endless paddy fields and swampy areas. Vung Tau was a big town with a busy port full of warships, patrol boats and cargo ships. It was an old French resort town and was a holiday location for wealthy Vietnamese from Saigon.

We arrived at the Badcoe Club, a modest building with louver windows that allowed the cool ocean breezes to waft through. Named after a Victoria Cross recipient, Peter Badcoe, the club was close to the beach. We passed in our rifles so they could be locked up in the armoury, a weight off our minds as we settled in to enjoy our break.

For the next couple of days, we went swimming at the nearby beach, had a few beers and watched movies at the Badcoe Club, checked out the bars along the congested streets of Vung Tau, where Aussie diggers and US servicemen were everywhere. Outside the bars were sexy young Vietnamese girls wearing miniskirts and hot pants, calling out and inviting us in for a drink.

"Eh, Uc-dai-loi (Aussie) ... you want me?" They called as we passed. "You buy me Saigon tea?" "You want number one boom boom?" "You, number one I give you fuck." As a 21-year-old, I was scared shitless and I resisted the temptation with my thoughts of the dreaded drip and other venereal diseases.

We also visited the Beachcomber Club at the American base. The base had a self-service store, gift shop, barber shop and a large cafeteria where we enjoyed lunch.

We returned to Nui Dat on the 23rd May at 1600 hours. It rained very heavily all the way and we all got soaking wet.

On the 6th June, 15 rockets exploded into Nui Dat. Most landed in the dump area and some crashed into the dirt of Luscombe airfield. The one that hit the hill was barely 200 metres away from my tent. I was on gun pit duty at the time and the rocket came within 70 metres of the Kanga Pad. Local towns and villages were also bombarded. The infantry and cavalry boys killed 45 VC, wounded two and took five prisoners while two Australians died and 17 were wounded. There was no respite. Another three rockets blasted into Nui Dat the following day wounding yet another Aussie soldier. We were placed on red alert.

On the same day I had to go out on a cipher run by Land Rover to 5 RAR on Operation Hammer near the small village of

Binh Ba about 5 kilometres away from Nui Dat to change their radio codes.

The Battle of Binh Ba (6–8 June 1969)

Two days later, 6 RAR was on patrol just outside the Nui Dat wire when there was a contact. Another digger died. I was on gun pit duty that evening from 2030 to 2230 hours, there was continuous gunfire from Nui Dat hill plus a lot of activity outside the wire as we set off flares.

It wasn't all bad news as I discovered I'd passed my Subject C (Army law) for corporal rank.

On Black Friday the 13th our squadron hosted a group of Tasmanian singers. We all dragged our deckchairs over to the open-air tent and enjoyed listening to the talented singers. Afterwards we had a barbeque.

Such a welcome relief from the daily routine and lifted our morale particularly the female singers.

The usual routine resumed the following day until Shorty Thompson went berserk in the canteen. I'd known Shorty since the School of Signals at Balcombe, and he worked with us in the ComCen as a signal delivery service driver. Shorty obviously had too much to drink on the night and started fighting with a few of the other signallers in the canteen, throwing a few objects around and upending deckchairs. The duty officer, Lieutenant Emery, kicked him out of the canteen and ordered him to go to his tent to sleep it off. Shorty did as he was told, but moments later, returned with a loaded rifle.

After threatening to shoot Emery, Shorty was overpowered and placed under arrest. Before he was charged, he went AWOL (Absent Without Leave) with another signaller and caught a lift in an Army truck from the main Nui Dat gates to Vung Tau. They were caught in Vung Tau, charged and sentenced to two weeks of detention in jail.

When the order came for someone to escort Shorty to the Australian Army jail in Vung Tau, I was nominated. The duty was tough as I was Shorty's mate. On the 24th June, Sig Bluey Baird and I escorted him to Vung Tau jail. Shorty was a skinny little bloke and he looked pale and nervous when we collected and drove him to Luscombe airfield. In preparation for the trip by Caribou, I had a pistol and carried Shorty's Army bag.

Our trip by Caribou to Vung Tau took 15 minutes and on our arrival at the airport two burly Military Policemen (Provosts) met us. The Provosts grabbed Shorty and pushed him into the back of a Land Rover. The jail or lock-up was known as 'The Hill' and was located on the side of a sand dune. It was a real eye-opener. Prisoners were mindlessly filling and emptying sandbags and running up and down the dune. I'd heard stories that some had to clean their cells with a toothbrush.

On our arrival at the jail, the Provosts removed our weapons and emptied Shorty's bag for inspection. After that, he was stripped naked.

"You'll regret you ever put your foot in these doors," one of the Provosts yelled at Shorty.

Shorty looked terrified and stood to attention, naked, white-faced and shaking as the burly Military Policeman ridiculed him.

To help take our minds off Shorty's fate we went for a swim

and a few beers at the Badcoe Club before catching a convoy back to Nui Dat.

> ***Shorty was having major problems back home. Along with the everyday pressure of stress and fatigue, his state of mind got the better of him and he lost the plot. This is a hallmark of PTSD. I was upset for weeks and to this day I cannot believe how the Provosts ridiculed and humiliated him while naked in front of us. Shorty was never the same when he returned to our unit. He seemed disconnected to us all.***

It was relatively quiet at Nui Dat. However, that all changed on 26th June when four rockets hit us at 0020 hours. I was asleep at the time, but soon leapt out of bed as they flew low over the base making a distinctive swooshing and whistling sound. I dived into our pit hole as they exploded and I remained there for an hour while the US artillery fired continuously over our heads. Two rockets landed 70 metres away and a couple more exploded by 6 RAR before the all-clear was given.

The following day Major Morel informed me of my impending promotion to Corporal. My morale lifted as I'd achieved something significant. I was only 21 years old.

High priority messages always required urgent delivery to the infantry, the artillery or one of the other armoured regiments. In the daytime, we used a signal delivery service driver to take the message, but at night it was a different story with no delivery service driver on duty. As shift leader I was responsible to deliver the message myself but with restricted movements at night, I had to seek permission from the Task Force Headquarters. They would only permit it if there was sufficient light as headlights were not allowed.

I dreaded these trips as without headlights, navigating on the roads was difficult and dangerous especially driving near manned gun pits. I was always worried someone would have a shot at us, thinking we were the VC. Often flares would go off as we passed by the gun pits.

Often, I noticed and heard a noisy machine go by my tent. It was a device on the back of a Land Rover. The machine was pumping out some obscure chemical shit into the barbed-wire area between the Kanga Pad and our signal lines. The stench from the spray drifted into my tent and forced me out.

The use of chemicals was widespread. When I was at FSB Julia and Kerry the Americans would fly over the nearby jungle area and spray defoliation chemicals. Often the spray drifted into the Fire Support Bases and it smelt something awful. I had no idea what it was but years later in 1978 when the Australian press first reported the effects of Agent Orange on soldiers, the Australian Government denied its use. Soon thousands of cases emerged.

In July my eyes were still troubling me. Sensitive to the humidity and dust, my eyelids were always red, my eyes perpetually bloodshot. It made me look even more exhausted than I was. I visited the RAP again, and the doctor gave me more antibiotic eye drops and ointment and instructed me to wash my eyes a couple of times a day in warm, salty water.

I often wonder if this was an effect of Agent Orange.

In July it rained hard almost every day. Monsoonal weather was typically hot and humid. I was hoping the monsoon season was almost over as the rain brought out little flying bugs in full force. The little buggers were everywhere, particularly at night with our tent lights on. The most annoying time was when you were having something to eat or drink, and they landed in your mouth. Mildew was another problem. Clothes in cupboards and bags were the worst affected. After surveying the damage, I discovered that many of my clothes had succumbed including my beret and slouch hat, resulting in me throwing them out knowing that the Q Store would replace them.

On the 14th July, Red Cross nurses visited us. They gave us each a parcel containing pens, writing pads, chocolate bars and a few toiletries.

Their kindness was a welcome gift that made us feel we were not forgotten.

At the beginning of August, the VC blew up a bridge on the road to Vung Tau. The bridge lay on a strategic route and straddled swamp and marshlands, and the disruption saw military and civilian traffic backed up for kilometres. The VC had done a good job with the old bridge, blowing it clean in half and forcing the Australian engineers to erect a temporary pontoon. This disrupted our trips to Vung Tau.

At the same time, the VC fired rockets into Baria, a small town ten kilometres from Nui Dat killing three civilians and wounding several others.

Incidents like this were normal stuff for us, and you knew you couldn't dwell on them. You just had to get on with it.

It was particularly busy in the Signal Centre/ComCen during the first couple of weeks in August. Operators handled outgoing messages every seven minutes and dealt with incoming messages every two minutes. On the switchboard, calls came in every seven seconds. I was currently working 80.5 hours over nine days in the Signal Centre, not counting cipher runs or gun pit duties.

Having been promoted Corporal at the end of July, I started on a Subject 'C' course for Sergeant for two hours daily. The course would proceed until November 22. It was going to be a busy time juggling coursework with the demands of the Signal Centre, cipher runs and gun pit duties.

At times on cipher runs I had trouble getting transport. In mid-August I boarded a Sioux 'Possum' chopper for another cipher run, taking the passenger seat. The pilot handed me some earphones and we took off. No sooner were we in the air when he received a message from the Task Force requesting he undertake some surveillance work for the infantry. With a lot of VC activity in the area, the pilot had no option but to drop me off at the nearest Fire Support Base. At the FSB I leapt out of the chopper and headed to the headquarter's tent. Unable to change the sets at the other bases, I contacted Jock Bannigan who suggested I get a lift back with an in-coming chopper. No choppers landed all day. Increasingly concerned I might be spending the night, I went to find the Duty Officer in the headquarter's tent. "No choppers available, Corporal. All being used by the infantry. You're not the only one trying to get back, you know," the Duty Officer replied.

I resigned myself to staying the night without a pit hole, and with artillery field batteries booming all night. To my relief, just before dusk an American Iroquois chopper arrived with a General and his aides on board. The Duty Officer asked if they could take a few Aussies back to Nui Dat. Minutes later, four of us scrambled aboard. There was limited space, and I was ordered to share a seat with an American gunner on the left side of the chopper. As the chopper took off and veered to the left trying to gain height, I gripped my rifle in one hand and the plunger bag in the other as the chopper swept in huge circles and gradually gained altitude. The dust below and around us swirled in huge, billowing clouds. I had my hands full and felt unstable. The gunner leant across and yelled above the noise. "Hey man, do you think you're going to fall out?"

"Yes, mate, I do," I yelled in reply.

"You won't fall out, man. You're like water in a whirling bucket. Water never falls out, man."

I nodded, though I still contemplated that he might be wrong as the chopper finally straightened out and headed back to Nui Dat. In the distance I could see pockets of artillery gunfire. Fifteen minutes later, and much to my relief, the four of us scrambled out onto the Kanga Pad. Seconds later, the chopper headed back to Vung Tau and we waved to the departing Yanks.

On 21st August 5 RAR stumbled into another VC bunker system. One digger killed and 34 more had been wounded in the incident. l sent reports out on the casualties. I realised what a hard time 5 RAR was experiencing.

In the middle of September, I was on another cipher run. I was heading to a Fire Support Base in a convoy of ten vehicles when there was an almighty boom followed by a shower of metal fragments as a wheel from the tip truck landed 50 metres away. Our truck skidded to a halt and I instantly flung myself onto the floorboards at the back of the truck while another couple of diggers jumped off into a nearby ditch at the side of the dirt road. I would have followed them, but I was loaded with gear including my rifle, a locked satchel with dispatches and a radio key plunger. I was about 100 metres away from the blast, but there was plenty of chaos, panic and confusion. Most of us thought it was an ambush, but as there was only one explosion, we soon realised it was a landmine. Two American soldiers died. We were stuck on the road for hours like sitting ducks wondering if, or rather, when the VC would attack. Once the Australian engineers swept the road with mine detectors and cleared a landing area for the dust-off chopper, we were on the move again.

> ***The incident scared the living hell out of me, particularly at night over the subsequent weeks as I tried to sleep but my brain, mind, thoughts and dreams constantly relived the tragic scene. The incident still haunts me with PTSD symptoms.***

In the last week of September, I headed to Vung Tau for the day along with a few other signallers. We visited the crowded market and were shocked at the lack of hygiene at the food stalls. Thousands of flies hovered over meat and fish or anything edible they could find. We walked through the market stalls, being waylaid by dozens of Vietnamese children wanting handouts or trying to sell us cheap souvenirs. They had trays around their necks and were selling cigarette lighters, flick knives, sunglasses and cigarette packets which we discovered contained marijuana sticks. We were cautious, knowing the children had reputations as excellent pickpockets. As we walked along the busy streets, a mob of kids soon gathered around, pulling and tugging at our uniforms. "Uc-dai-loi buy," they yelled in unison, urging us to buy souvenirs. We pushed them away, but they responded by yelling even louder. "Uc-dai-loi Cheap Charlie, Uc-dai-loi Cheap Charlie."

There must have been a dozen of them ranging in ages from six to twelve, slightly built with long slender legs and arms. Until then, I hadn't realised their strength as I struggled to hang onto my precious camera. We moved on, and I later realised that I'd lost $40 in military payment certificates. It must have been pilfered by one of the kids. I had been warned and was thankful my camera had survived. We reported the incident to the South Vietnamese Police who were known as White Mice, not only because they wore white shirts, but also for their attitude under fire. They were not interested in my lost money, obviously had more pressing matters to deal with.

I received a letter from friends, Mr and Mrs Stiensen, informing me that Mum was not well. I decided to go home on R&R (Rest and Recreation) instead of Hong Kong.

Well overdue for a break, I knew that, over the past few weeks, even small inconsequential things had been starting to annoy me. Either I lost my patience and became irritable or became depressed and apathetic for days. I'd been in Vietnam for 265 days, a lifetime for me. Home was like an elusive dream, always just out of reach.

On the morning of 28th September, I boarded the Caribou. The trip to Saigon took half an hour, but we were delayed for another half an hour due to fog. I had eight hours to spare, leaving for home at 1730 hours. To fill in time, I caught an American forces bus from the airport into Saigon and took a rickshaw ride around Saigon visiting the main sights, including monuments and statues, wealthy suburbs criss-crossed by tree-lined boulevards and spacious French colonial mansions surrounded by lush tropical gardens and on to the city's commercial hub with its brightly coloured bars, clubs and sidewalk cafes. The place was incredibly noisy and feverish with bicycles, Lambrettas, rickshaws, motor scooters, cars and buses cluttering the streets and emitting a haze of exhaust fumes.

With a full roll of film, I headed back to Tan Son Nhut airport and departed on time at 1730 hours with a full plane of noisy American and Australian servicemen to Brisbane via Darwin and Sydney.

> *It was a very emotional feeling coming home. I felt strange to be in a peaceful place again and although Vietnam was twelve hours away by air, the Vietnam War was plastered on the front pages of every newspaper headlines in the country as well as radio and television. I couldn't get away from the place and I soon discovered how the topic of the Vietnam war came up in conversation with lots of anti-war demonstrations going on all over Australia. I rested, surfed at Kings Beach and enjoyed Mum's cooking for my five days of R&R but in the end, it was a big mistake coming home as time passed too quickly and it was hard to say goodbye all over again. Maybe if I had spent my leave in Hong Kong it would have been easier on everyone. I found this goodbye*

much harder than when I had first left for Vietnam – thinking about the place I was returning to with my mind swirling with images of death and destruction.

Back at hot steamy Nui Dat nothing had changed – it felt as if I'd never been away. My R&R evaporated like a dream, and I was back in the God-forsaken stinking joint. The only consolation was I had only 100 days left in Vietnam before I would be home for good.

My days were soon filled with shift duty in the Signal Centre and cipher runs to forward elements. I detested cipher runs especially after my near miss in mid-September when I witnessed two American soldiers killed by a landmine while travelling in a convoy to a fire support base. The more of these runs I completed, the more fear I experienced.

Travelling in the two-man Sioux helicopter was a scary experience. The pilot flew at treetop level and low over small fishing villages and jungle areas to avoid the VC having time to get a shot at us. As passengers we acted as observers for any VC activity on the ground. Pilots were highly skilled and had nerves of steel in controlling the small choppers, particularly when we experienced shock waves from artillery guns, ground explosions and enemy fire plus all the steep landings and take-offs. On these runs I would carry a revolver rather than an SLR as the cockpit was too small. On the larger Iroquois choppers or road convoys, I always had my rifle. On all cipher runs I also carried a locked satchel with top secret signal dispatches along with the radio key plunger.

By mid-October I was on night shift. One night a Signal Delivery Service driver came into the Signal Centre in the early hours of the morning drunk and disorderly. He grabbed a stack of mail including a bag of letters and couple of parcels. "Gordon, what are you doing with that mail, mate?" I yelled.

Another signaller and I followed him into the darkness. In his drunken stupor, the driver emptied the bag and parcels down the shit hole of the toilet block.

> ***I knew he was under pressure and was reluctant to charge him. However, the Cipher Sergeant and the Troop Sergeant handed me the report all ready for my signature. A few days later I marched the driver into Major Morel's office, where he was formally charged. He received fourteen days confined to barracks (CB).***

Early in November our squadron conducted ambush patrols outside the main wire at Nui Dat. I was instructed to go on one, it would be my first ambush patrol. I had been on lots of clearing patrols at Fire Support Bases. I had to meet the other members of the patrol outside our Headquarters building at 1500 hours with all my gear for a briefing.

I fronted up, I discovered there were 12 of us on the patrol including two Sergeants with one of them to carry the radio on his back. Apart from myself as Corporal, there were eight other Signallers and a Medic who I hadn't met before.

The plan was to set up an ambush five kilometres from the Nui Dat wire on a narrow track in a clearing close to dense jungle foliage. We moved out late that afternoon by truck and were dropped a couple of kilometres down the road. Soon we were moving in single file, four to six metres apart, in the stifling heat. I was loaded with my webbing gear, including water canteens, ration pack, full magazines, rifle, bayonet and ammunition belts around my shoulder for the machine-gun. The machine-gun was carried by another patrol member. My greens were quickly saturated, my face running in rivulets of sweat.

We reached the ambush site around dusk. After setting up the area with Claymore mines and trip flares, we gulped our ration packs. We were on the edge of the jungle facing an open area and the track along which we'd just walked. We were instructed to stay awake and alert for the rest of the night.

The first few hours passed quickly. My adrenalin was running high as I listened to every creaking jungle sound in the damp air and sticky earth. Noises magnified as the night went on and I started imagining things. With the dampness of my jungle greens and clammy skin, I felt like scratching myself all over and had aching cramps in my body from being in one position for too long. Soon I was fighting fatigue, struggling to keep my eyes open as my concentration dropped. I'd nod off then jerk awake, and realise I was in the middle of the stinking Vietnamese jungle. This was repeated all night until the sun rose, and I heaved a sigh of relief that the VC hadn't wandered down the track during the night. After disarming the Claymores and trip flares, we made our way back to Nui Dat.

It was still early November. I had fewer than 60 days plus a wakey to serve in country. Time was passing quickly. I was sitting in my tent when a Public Relations Officer appeared. He asked me if I wanted to send a Christmas message to my family and friends back in Caloundra by voice tape, I agreed. The PR man recorded a short message.

It was such a comforting thought that my message along with those of many others would be played on radio station 4IP on Christmas Day.

In the early hours of the morning on 8th November, the noise of choppers landing and taking off woke me. I poked my head out the tent flap and peered through the barbed wire and watched them for a few minutes as they came in to refuel. Tanks and APCs were grinding along the road near the Kanga Pad heading towards the main gate. Later, I learnt that a large contingent of VC had attacked Long Dien, a small Observation Post around eight kilometres from Nui Dat. A few South Vietnamese soldiers had been killed, and the Australian officer wounded.

The post was abandoned. I had been to Long Dien many times on cipher runs to change their radio set codes.

The remainder of November was busy for me with shift work in the Signal Centre and completing a subject course for Sergeant which took two weeks.

In the last week of November, a 'Safe Hand' package containing captured documents was delivered to the Signal Centre. The package was addressed to Major General Hay, the Commander of Australian Forces in Vietnam. The Intelligence Officer instructed me to put the package on the first flight going to Saigon. I ordered our duty driver to take the package to the aircraft in the Safe Handbag. It was never delivered. It was later found under a pile of mail waiting to be sorted. As I was responsible, having been on duty at the time I was charged with negligence by Captain Horne and Warrant Officer Jock

Bannigan. When I returned to duty next evening, I asked our duty driver why he hadn't delivered the parcel. The driver made some lame excuse saying he didn't know anything about the package. When he offered me his fists, I responded by charging him with two counts of offering violence.

The following day I was marched into Major Morel's office, formally charged with neglect and received a reprimand. He told me to be more careful, more alert and to ensure I did thorough checks of any Safe Hand articles in future. The Signal Delivery Service driver was fined $30 and given seven days field punishment for threatening violence based on evidence from my four witnesses.

Whenever we travelled on the roads outside Nui Dat, particularly dirt roads and those that were less busy, we had to be wary of landmines. A quarter of all the Australians killed in Vietnam died as a result of mines and booby traps. On most convoys we had Engineer sappers up front on APCs looking for anything suspicious. The instant they suspected something, the convoy would stop, and the engineer would clear the road with a mine detector. On one occasion our convoy came across a car blown up by a landmine. The driver was dead in a heartbeat and I was instantly transported back to when an American Army tip truck hit a landmine killing two American soldiers.

A few days later and on a more positive note, I received news of having passed Subject 'C' for Sergeant.

On the 7th December to 12th December I went on my R&C leave (Rest and Convalescence) to Vung Tau with another Signaller, Derek (Dick) Stainer, a Switchboard Operator. We stayed at the R&C centre, slept in every morning and went to the beach for a swim, or walked over to the Badcoe Club pool where we'd laze about in the sun and enjoy a few drinks. We also visited the American Beachcomber Club and went on a few tours of Vung Tau enjoying the wide boulevard-style streets, and the lively local markets. In the evenings, we mostly watched movies.

It was a relief to be away from the stress of the cipher runs that always had me on edge.

I will never forget my last work party. I was rostered on to do the water and garbage run using a Land Rover and trailer around our lines, to pick up all the rubbish bins including the wet garbage scraps from the kitchen and dump them at the rubbish tip. After this we were expected to complete the water run by switching trailers to a tank trailer, driving to the water station and filling the tank trailer plus other containers before returning to our lines to deliver water to various locations.

One of my shift workers, a 'Nasho', Signaller Graeme Stevens, was rostered on with me. Stevo as we all called him was a friendly bloke, a farmer from Gawler in South Australia. You could never tell whether he was serious or joking because his face had a perpetual smirk. The South Australian made it plain he didn't like being in the Army. Pissed off when he got called up for National Service, Stevo was always grumbling about the Army and the government. He reckoned it would have been better for him to remain a farmer and grow food for the country.

At the Kanga Pad gate next to our lines, Stevo and I picked up the last rubbish bin before we were ready to head to the tip. The gate was next to an open-roofed shelter which was a passenger waiting area for the choppers. Waiting in the shelter were half a dozen Australian and American Army top brass officers in crisp green Army uniforms and shiny boots. Stevo and I must have looked scruffy in our sweaty greens.

"Look at those fucking big brass bastards in their fucking clean uniforms. They wouldn't know how to get their hands dirty," Stevo muttered. We grabbed the heavy drum full of rubbish and lifted it to the back trailer, and I instructed Stevo to drive to the tip.

We got into the Land Rover, and Stevo put his foot down. There was a screeching as the wheels burned-off followed by a clonk as the last two drums on the trailer tumbled onto the bitumen, one of them full of wet garbage scraps. The rubbish splattered in all directions including on the shiny boots and the lower legs of the uniformed officers. Stevo stopped the Land Rover, and I looked back.

"Idiots!" the officers yelled, "Where's your brains?"

I felt like running away, especially when one of the officers walked up to the driver's door.

"And you can get that smirk off your face, Private, or I will charge you," he yelled inches from Stevo's face.

"What's your unit, Corporal?" another yelled, "Get this mess cleaned up straight away!"

Fortunately for us, the chopper landed, and the crew signalled to the top brass to get aboard. It certainly saved our backsides as we watched six deflated high-ranking officers trudge despondently through the wet slush towards the chopper. Stevo was elated, although it took us half an hour to clean up the mess as we shovelled the muck into the bin accompanied by thousands of resident flies.

CHAPTER 9

GETTING SHORT

I had two weeks left to serve in country. On Christmas Eve I began my RTA (return to Australia) 'happy' pills. Before returning to Australia we were given Primaquine and Chloroquine tablets to help clear up any malaria or bugs in our system.

On Christmas Day, frustratingly I copped the day shift from 0800 hours to 1600 hours.

With the main celebrations taking place in the mess from midday onwards, we decided to split the shifts, so everyone had a chance to celebrate for an hour. There was an excellent Christmas spread with turkey, chicken, cold ham, vegetables, ice-cream and tinned fruit. Christmas tradition dictated that officers and sergeants served the diggers. After 1600 hours, we all got stuck in and enjoyed the festive atmosphere.

I was crook for a couple of days after Christmas due to the RTA pills with vomiting and diarrhoea.

Tuesday 6th January 1970 was my last day at Nui Dat. I cleared out my rubbish and returned my Army gear including my rifle and webbing to the Squadron Store.

That evening the squadron put on a going home party for Richard Burgess and me in the boozer. It felt good to be the hub of the celebration. I made a speech and was presented with a pewter tankard engraved with my name and squadron. Filled with beer I toasted my return and dutifully sculled every drop. After the boozer closed, we went to our respective tents to continue celebrating.

After midnight, when everyone left, I had a final cold shower. I knew my next shower would be a warm one. I dropped into bed, but I couldn't sleep as I tossed and turned for the rest of the night from sheer excitement.

Next morning, 7th January, dressed in my polyester uniform I clambered aboard the Hercules at Luscombe airfield along with Richard Burgess for our flight to Saigon.

Half an hour later, we landed at Tan Son Nhut airport and I saw the Qantas 707 Freedom Bird waiting on the tarmac, to take me home.

I remember being filled with excitement and anticipation about going home.

It was such a wonderful sight, and I had a lump in my throat knowing it symbolised my future.

We boarded the Freedom Bird and I sat next to Richard Burgess and Bill Scott, a tank driver who I'd last seen amid the mayhem at FSB Julia. I couldn't help thinking how ironic it was that the three of us who had finished rookie training together at Kapooka were now returning home together. The plane taxied along the runway then made a steep ascent and everyone cheered as we left Vietnam behind. Soon, the mountains of Long Hai were obliterated by cloud. I relaxed back in my seat and thought about all the good and bad times I'd had in Vietnam, about my future and getting home to my family.

Diggers were playing cards, reading, chatting but were mostly just sitting and staring, absorbed in their own thoughts or sleeping. I slept most of the way to Sydney before we landed at Mascot after midnight to a rousing cheer from the diggers as we finally touched down on Australian soil. We disembarked into a huge hangar some distance away from the main terminal, and several diggers dropped to their knees and kissed the ground.

We were quickly processed through Customs. It was an emotional time as loved ones greeted one another, wives, girlfriends, family and friends hugging and kissing with lots of tears. Scotty and I said goodbye to Richard who was off to somewhere in Sydney while we took a taxi to an expensive hotel in the city. It was hot and humid.

We arrived at the hotel and I asked the clerk for two rooms. At the same time, some American tourists arrived, and the clerk asked us to step aside as he had more important work to do than serving us, while he served them. We were both stunned and speechless. If we hadn't been so tired, we would have told the clerk where to stick it. However, worn down by travel, we couldn't be bothered and waited patiently in line still processing the fact that we were finally home.

CHAPTER 10

BACK HOME

We arrived at our rooms in the early hours of the morning. After I enjoyed my first hot shower in months, my head hit the pillow and I was immediately asleep. When my eyes opened at 0630 hours I'd slept through the alarm and had to rebook my ticket to Brisbane.

Scotty and I caught a taxi from the hotel to the airport. A group of anti-Vietnam war demonstrators had gathered outside the terminal and were waving placards protesting the war. When we emerged from the taxi, the demonstrators saw our uniforms and rushed towards us, yelling foul language. They called us baby killers and shouted that we should both be in jail.

The Anti-War Demonstrations

The My Lai Massacre occurred on 16 March 1968 and was carried out by American Army soldiers in Vietnam. Between 347 and 504 unarmed civilians were killed including men,

women, children and infants. Some of the women were gang raped. The story broke in the media on 12 November 1969 while I was still serving in Vietnam.

When I returned home, the scornful words 'baby killers' were written on placards with prominent photos of the bodies of dead babies while screaming anti-war protestors yelled 'baby killers' and threw pig blood at us as a response to the inhumanity of the massacre.

This was not our sin, and yet it would be used to taint our service, and to dishonour my time in Vietnam.

Scotty and I made our way to the terminal with the demonstrators jostling and heckling us, making us feel uncomfortable. When we reached the main doors, a young woman lunged towards me. A glob of spit hit my left cheek. I dropped my bags and wiped my face, fuming and shaking from the incident.

"Can you believe this? The bitch spat on me! This is all shit." I said to Scotty.

"I know, Morg. They're a bloody bunch of commos and hippies. If you ask me, they should all be put away. They hate the sight of our uniform. That's why the government brings us back after midnight to avoid pricks like them," Scotty yelled.

I went to wash my face and hands in the men's toilets before we headed to the check-in-desk. Scotty was leaving on an earlier flight to Melbourne. My flight to Brisbane left on time and landed on schedule later that morning. My welcome home wasn't as emotional as it had been three months before, but nevertheless it was wonderful to see my family.

I felt a sense of satisfaction, but also some confusion, particularly when we were confronted with more anti-Vietnam

War demonstrators outside the terminal. I felt like a criminal. The demonstrators were holding placards with slogans such as 'Peace not War' and 'Australia get out of Vietnam'. Thankfully, they were not as aggressive as those in Sydney.

> *It was a rude shock to return home 'under fire'. While I never expected a hero's welcome, I never thought that, while being away striving under our nation's flag, I would have earned such disrespect from our civilian countrymen and women. It was a bitter pill to swallow. The labels of 'brute', 'murderer', 'child killer' and 'warmonger' were cruel and untrue. I had done my job but earned notoriety.*
>
> *It took me a long time to reconcile the fact that I had just worked my guts out, faced night after night of gut-wrenching fear, and lived in a hovel for nothing, in fact, for less than nothing. I'd wasted a year of my life in appalling conditions, not to mention the threat to my own life. I'd gained nothing, lost the respect and friendship of people I knew. I had been fighting for freedom, democracy and for my country Australia – how could that have been wrong?*
>
> *To my amazement, in many ways I didn't want to be home. I wanted to be alone or back in Vietnam. It was a strange feeling, to feel so distant from other people, even mates I'd known for years. I was consumed with anger within myself and further fuelled by watching the negative bullshit from politicians as well as the ranting of peace demonstrators on TV.*
>
> *Even my mum noticed I had dramatically changed from being soft-natured and carefree before Vietnam into an emotionless, cold person with bursts of anger and coarse language on my return. I was like a stranger to all my family.*

I believe coming home to a deeply hostile reception and lack of social support contributed a higher level of my PTSD symptoms.

For the next month on leave, I relaxed and caught waves at Kings Beach. I decided to buy a car with the $3000 I'd saved. I scoured the second-hand dealers and finally settled on a 1968 Holden Torana HB for just over $2000.

On my last week of leave, I received a registered package containing my War Medals. I thought the medals were always presented on the Parade Ground.

I was furious, I felt like throwing my medals out. This ploy by the Australian government was cheap, disrespectful and disgraceful.

CHAPTER 11

MY FINAL POSTINGS IN THE ARMY

I finished my leave early February and was posted to 4 Signal Regiment at Wacol on the Ipswich Highway west of Brisbane. My work time was divided between the busy Signal Centre at Victoria Barracks in the heart of Brisbane, and the one-man operation at Wacol Signal Centre.

It was a horrible time to be in the Armed Forces or wearing a uniform and having short hair as it often identified me as a soldier. I was reluctant to wear my uniform outside the barracks, but it was impossible when I was working at Victoria Barracks. I had to go down to a nearby café in my uniform to buy meals while on shift duty. I always tried to avoid the ugly demonstrators but often people would look at me in a distasteful manner. One fellow shift worker returned from the city upset and shaken when he was chased by abusive demonstrators and felt his life so threatened that he took refuge in a barber's shop and asked the barber to cover his uniform up with a cape (a barber's sleeveless garment).

With this social hatred I felt like a common criminal.

At Victoria Barracks I was busy all the time while at Wacol I sat on my backside bored shitless. I was torn between two worlds, one of boredom and the other utterly chaotic.

The living conditions at Wacol were atrocious. I was housed in an old wooden building with a dormitory set-up of four beds on one side and four on the other, each separated by large metal lockers. At each end of the building were the toilets, showers and washrooms. People coming in late interrupted everyone else's sleep by walking on creaky boards or banging the door of their metal locker. If those disturbances didn't wake you, the mosquitoes certainly did.

I was only at Wacol for two weeks when some thieving bastard knocked off my Vietnam-issued Army trunk. I'd put the trunk under my bed and padlocked it. Inside the trunk, I had some valuable gear I'd purchased from the Yanks in Vietnam such as an American flak jacket, American unit badges, a pair of American Army boots, uniform and cap. There were also some of my own items including a machete, new issued Army greens and boots plus some personal papers including movement papers and air tickets to Vietnam. I reported the theft to the Commanding Officer who seemed uninterested. He told me I should have left the trunk at home or chained it to my bed.

I was pissed off and angry.

In early May, on my request, I transferred back to my former unit, 139 Signal Squadron at Enoggera Army Barracks. This was a field unit where I could get out into the bush on exercises rather than being indoors. At the squadron, I was one of a handful of soldiers who had been to Vietnam. The rest of the squadron were new to the Army.

Although I felt a lot happier in my old unit, in July 1970, after three years in the Army, I elected to be discharged.

For the past couple of months, I'd questioned whether Army life was for me. Increasingly, I found everything in the Army to be negative, and I knew the media was playing a big part by broadcasting adverse stories of our involvement in Vietnam.

Wherever I went, I felt the disapproval of the Army, Vietnam War and National Service. Even within our own ranks, I found negativity towards the Army, particularly from the Nashos pissed off from being called up and serving.

My decision shocked everyone. Most thought I was a lifer. My Commanding Officer tried to talk me round, promising me a bright future and promotion to Sergeant by the end of the year. The possibility of promotion didn't sway my decision. I needed to take control of my life. Ever since returning from Vietnam, I'd felt unsettled. I told my Commanding Officer that the fact that people did not recognise the service I'd given to my country played on my mind, and I felt I'd lost my ability to enjoy life, I'd become too sensitive and serious. I admitted that I'd miss the Army, particularly the mateship and comradeship. However, my mind was made up.

It was a young Army officer who finally helped make up my mind. This officer was in charge of our troop, and one Friday afternoon there was an inspection of our lines. I was in charge of our troop lines. The young Lieutenant, just out of the Royal Military College at Duntroon, inspected our rooms, showers, toilets and laundry blocks. He wasn't too impressed with the cleanliness, neatness and standards of our rooms, and ordered another inspection at 2000 hours. As it was Friday afternoon, we were all eager to get away for the weekend.

At the next inspection, we once again failed. When the Lieutenant ordered the next inspection for 0900 hours Saturday morning, I questioned his attitude. Was he pissed off because he was the Duty-Officer for the weekend? Surely, he wouldn't call an inspection if he had the weekend off. At every inspection, he would pick up trivial things. The inspections continued until midday Saturday when he finally passed the troop. I could see his little mind games at work. My impression of him was that he thought he was a god-like officer, superior to everyone else, a total control freak. That was the final straw, and I decided Army life was not for me.

CHAPTER 12

CIVILIAN LIFE

I wanted to return to flying and applied to an aviation flying school in NSW to get my Commercial Pilot's Licence. I decided to take a few refresher lessons at Maroochydore airport with my old flying instructor but sadly found it impossible to get into the small Cessna 150. As soon as the doors were closed, I was overwhelmed with anxiety. I felt trapped and was reliving my pit hole incident at FSB Julia.

Unknown to me at the time, I was experiencing my first PTSD symptom of Anxiety with a sense of unreality. My breathing increased, heart rate increased, there was excessive sweating, blurry vision, butterflies in my stomach and my whole body was shaking. I felt like I was suffocating and going to die. I tried to explain to my flying instructor, but I don't think he understood what I was experiencing. As a result, I put my flying career on ice. I was still unsure whether I'd made the right decision by leaving the Army.

CHAPTER 12

One part of me wanted to find another life and another part pushed me to stay with my mates and serve my country.

Mum was shocked when I left the Army. However, I soon applied for various allied communications jobs with the Department of Civil Aviation, Foreign Affairs, Defence Signals and Department of Supply. I didn't confine myself to jobs I knew how to do. I also applied to work on an oil rig, and as a TV cameraman. The Department of Supply was the first to offer me a job in Melbourne at its high security Signal Centre. After I passed a Commonwealth police check for the job, I started in August 1970.

The Signal Centre had twelve Operators working five different circuits to London, Washington, Salisbury in South Australia, Sydney, Canberra and Army Melbourne. I handled messages, including top secret ones about supplies relating to the Australian Defence Force. I worked two shifts, two weeks on day, and one week on night shift. I found a respectable boarding house in East St Kilda. The accommodation was a single room, basic and clean. There were ten other boarders, all males, mainly apprentices or university students.

Weeks and months passed, and I became increasingly unsettled in my career and lifestyle.

I soon found myself battling nightmares and lack of sleep. I'd wake in a sweat, screaming out, gasping for breath and scrambling for the light switch. It felt like I was suffocating and dying in the pit hole back in Vietnam.

Sleep problems and nightmares are another PTSD symptom. With my nightmare I was re-experiencing my

> *traumatic event in Vietnam. I was "on alert" or "guard" all the time for danger and threat. As a result, I found it very difficult to fall asleep and to stay asleep. I was stuck in survival mode.*

My Vietnam mate, Robert 'Scotty' Wilson, was killed in Vietnam on 16th July 1971 on his second tour. I was shattered by the news. Scotty was only 21 years old, and his death was a profound loss to me. After Scotty's death, I became consumed with guilt. I felt guilty about leaving the Army and letting down my mates. A lot of anti-Vietnam War demonstrations and marches were taking place in Melbourne at the time, and I became angry and disgusted at their behaviour. All I wanted to do was to get out of Melbourne.

> *The Vietnam Moratorium marches were in full force at the time led by Dr Jim Cairns and swelled by the clergy, teachers, university professors, the unions, politicians – mainly Labour – and university students all opposed to the war and rallied to the ideal of 'peace'. The collision of war and peace literally split the nation with families, marriages and friends torn apart.*

I applied for jobs with the Army, the Bureau of Meteorology and Foreign Affairs. The Army said they would take me back with my rank and trade. The Bureau of Meteorology offered me a job in communications in either Melbourne or Darwin. I chose the Bureau job in Darwin. I liked the idea of a new job in a new environment with new challenges. I felt with the Army, I'd been there and done that, and I wanted to give civilian life more of a chance.

A couple months before I made the decision to leave Melbourne, I had met my first love, Jan Pratt, from Chelsea in Melbourne. Jan was a pretty, soft-natured, loving girl in her final year at high school, Year 12. When we went out on a few dates, I discovered my emotions were all mixed up. I wasn't even sure if I still had any feelings left as I was never able to express my true feelings towards Jan. I was having nightmares and felt confused and anxious most of the time.

> ***PTSD symptoms can cause negative impact on your relationships such as trust, closeness and communications. I found I couldn't share my thoughts and feelings with Jan and avoided talking about my problems. This was the same with my family and friends. I couldn't explain my behaviour, so I moved on.***

I started my new job early in January 1972, but soon discovered that Darwin was not the place for me. While I enjoyed the Bureau immensely, I struggled with the Darwin lifestyle. I lived at the Commonwealth Hostel on the Esplanade with other public servants, but I didn't have much in common with them. I kept company with the Customs' guys, some of whom were ex-Army and my Bureau of Meteorology workmates.

In Darwin's tropical climate, the conjunctivitis I'd last suffered in Vietnam returned to haunt me with a vengeance. A local doctor prescribed me some antibiotic ointment, but the conjunctivitis persisted in both my eyes. I went to see an eye specialist and he advised me to leave the tropics as my eyes were sensitive to the heat and humidity.

I was angry when I moved to Darwin and my new lifestyle

didn't help me to manage depression and anger. It was a drinking culture with the population made up mainly with males, so I spent a lot of time in the pubs drinking.

> ***I started drinking alcohol to cope with my painful symptoms of PTSD such as my flashbacks and nightmares of Vietnam. By drinking I could tolerate my feelings of fear and improve my social confidence by connecting with other people.***

The Commonwealth Hostel had single and double-storey buildings. My room was in a single building containing 14 rooms, seven rooms on each side along a corridor.

The guy living next to me was an Air-Traffic Controller. He came across as a smartarse, a know-all, and he was the only bloke in the entire building who had a girlfriend. He would take her regularly to his room to have sex. The problem was that it was exceptionally noisy, with his girlfriend moaning, groaning and screaming out. The noise echoed through the building and upset many of the residents. You often heard guys yelling out "Shut the fuck up!" The noisy sex went on for weeks which interrupted everyone's sleep including mine until one night, I couldn't take it any longer and banged on his door. "If you don't shut up, I will bang your fucking heads in!" I was angry. I punched the door with my fist, and the entire door exploded. I could hardly believe my own strength. After that, there was no sound from the couple, not even a whimper. When the Hostel Manager arrived to investigate the following morning, I had to laugh. He was looking for a sledgehammer, not a swollen, bloodied fist. Thankfully, the couple moved somewhere else to have sex because I never heard them again.

That wasn't the only drama my anger caused during my time in Darwin. Another time, I was caught up in an ugly fight when one of the young guys in a nearby room yelled out for help. My neighbour had caught a burglar in his room knocking off some money and valuables. Three guys from nearby rooms, including me, came to his rescue. The thief was a well-built European who only spoke broken English. In the chaos, we decided to teach him a lesson by delivering our own justice and belted the living daylights out of him. I had a lot of anger just bubbling away, and it felt good throwing punches. The desperate and bloodied thief managed to escape, but not before he also threw a few punches. One landed right on top of my head and stunned me. I ended up in Darwin hospital for a few hours with concussion. The police arrived to question us but by then, the thief had vanished along with the evidence of what my uncontrolled anger could do.

> ***Anger is a common response to trauma and frequently occurs with PTSD. It is a fundamental part of natural survival instinct to either "fight" or "flee" from danger. In the first incident, being hyper-aroused, tense and irritable all the time I was triggered by the disruption of my sleep and personal space. The second incident was a natural response to help a person facing danger. With the arousal of my anger, I had the sense of being in charge of the situation and able to assert my power but my anger made it hard to think clearly and to evaluate the options. I became more aggressive and acted on impulse without considering the consequences of my behaviour.***

With the Bureau understanding my problem with my eyes, I

transferred to Brisbane in late June 1972. My new job was as a Weather Assistant in the Forecast Centre. I sent out forecasts, plotted synoptic charts, compiled weather charts and composed rainfall bulletins and maps. I enjoyed the work, and it was good to be back home and close to my family again. Life seemed to settle down although I still had issues relating to Vietnam from time to time. At this stage, I discovered that I couldn't talk to anyone, including my own family, about the war. My emotions where bubbling but I simply bundled them up and hid them away. The first sign that I wasn't holding up well, was when the Regional Director of Meteorology, Arch Shields, called me into his office early in 1973. He asked why I'd taken more sickies than anyone else. I told him I was suffering from nerves and anxiety after serving in Vietnam and was struggling with life. Arch was the first person who understood my predicament and associated feelings.

> ***Arch had served in the Air Force during World War II, and he had more understanding of Vietnam veterans than most other ex-servicemen. In contrast, the old diggers in the RSL would say, "What war was that, son? That wasn't a bloody war, and even if it was a war, you all bloody lost it."***

The second time I broke my silence was in New Zealand. In midwinter 1973, my twin brother Don, a mate, Stephen Smyth and I went on holiday to New Zealand for a couple of weeks. In Queenstown, on the South Island, we were invited to a party by a jockey. An Australian bloke at the party got pissed off and upset when Don, Stephen and I enticed away his three lady friends. He started mouthing off in a big way and became more and more unsociable as the night unfolded. "The only bloody decent Kiwi I ever met was a dead one in a body bag from Vietnam!" he yelled out.

His comments struck a sensitive note with me. I saw red and stood up and yelled back. "Why don't you bloody shut up and piss off so we can enjoy ourselves. Disgraceful coward prick!"

A flying fist came straight at me from the six-foot big-mouth arsehole of an Aussie. The lights went out, and there was a brawl that culminated with this bloke throwing the jockey through a large plate glass window. Fortunately, the jockey was a robust little bugger and despite the four-foot drop came back inside, grabbed his shotgun and threatened to shoot the Aussie arsehole. Not surprisingly in the face of imminent danger, the Aussie fled, and we never saw him again.

For my part I ended up with four stitches to my lip. To this day, I have a fat lip to remind me of my own angry aggressive outburst.

On Australia Day weekend in January 1974, my Army training came in handy when Cyclone Wanda crossed the coast 150 kilometres north of Brisbane. I worked 60 hours in a 72-hour stretch in the Forecast Centre when my fellow shift workers couldn't get to work because of the flooding caused by the heavy rain. This was the first time I'd worked such long hours without sleep since my Vietnam days with that old familiar feeling of pressure and coping with sleep deprivation.

At this stage I was still having nightmares, drinking heavily and having anger outbursts. In one incident I put my fist

through my mum's bedroom door after an argument. Any little issue would set me off. My life wasn't going anywhere. I was falling slowly into a big black hole of depression.

CHAPTER 13

OVERSEAS TO USA AND CANADA

A year later in early February 1975, and four years since I'd left the Army, I finally saved enough money to travel overseas. I flew to the USA and spent a week in both Los Angeles and San Francisco and then got a bus to Portland in Oregon to visit my sister Patsy, who had married an American. I discovered my sister was being bashed and assaulted by her second husband, although Patsy denied it. Her first husband had done likewise, and they divorced, splitting the four children, resulting in two boys going with their father and the eldest boy and the youngest, a girl, going with Patsy. The two children with Patsy were also neglected by her new husband. I went out and bought them food and clothing and pleaded with my sister to get out and go back home to Australia.

I felt Patsy was in denial and scared about becoming homeless and destitute. I wanted to report the domestic

violence to police but she pleaded with me not to interfere in her life.

I already wasn't coping with my issues and the whole situation with my sister sent me into a black hole of depression. I was trying to enjoy myself, but I lost interest in all activities except drinking. I couldn't cope and everything seemed out of control. At this time, I had repeated thoughts about suicide and had self-destructive urges.

After one month with my sister I travelled to Seattle and then onto Vancouver in Canada, where I stayed a couple of weeks and spent most of my time in bars.

I was excessively thinking worthless thoughts and reminiscing, pondering life, my past and my future. I worked out a plan to do myself in. It was to get a one-way ticket across Canada to Montreal in Quebec and somewhere along the trip at a rail siding to disembark and disappear into the cold freezing landscape and die peacefully.

I bought the one-way ticket for a single cabin to Montreal. It was about a four-day journey. Strangely my mood and outlook changed, and my negative thoughts disappeared as my journey got underway. I thought how stupid I was to think about doing myself in. Maybe my mood changed with the activity of travelling and distraction from my problems and my sister's.

Whatever it was I seemed to have more motivation, sense of control over my thinking and was excited with my trip across Canada.

I spent most of the time in the observation carriage looking at the beautiful Canadian countryside and playing card games. I met loads of characters on the trip, mainly young adventurers like me who were travelling for vastly different reasons.

It was an awesome journey and a most enjoyable way to cross Canada. I was fully immersed in seeing the diverse landscape and large cities on my journey.

I didn't stay long in Montreal, only a couple of days. I found it hard to get around in the city with most people speaking only French. I then travelled by bus to the Big Apple, New York city, where I simply couldn't comprehend the number of people who lived and worked there. I'd never seen so many people in my life. I did all the touristy things such as going to the Statue of Liberty, Empire State building, New York Stock Exchange and the United Nations Headquarters and stood in awe at the Twin Towers of the World Trade Centre as they reached 110 storeys. Finally, I visited Central Park, an oasis of lakes, immaculately kept grass, beautiful mature trees and recreation facilities in the middle of the roar and bustle of the city.

I was in New York for a week and on the night of 30th April 1975, I flicked on the TV to watch the fall of Saigon and the end of the Vietnam War. It was a strange, painful feeling watching people scrambling into helicopters in a desperate attempt to escape the communists, and helicopters being ditched in the sea from an American aircraft carrier.

I turned the TV off, unable to control the volatile emotions I was experiencing. I headed down to the bar of the hotel to get drunk. My thinking: 'What a waste of lives and time it had been'. The drinking helped me to block out bad memories from Vietnam, but it was only a short relief for my anger and

> ***depression. At the bar I came across a small scrap of paper with Ron Casey's name and address in my wallet. As I sat at the bar memories flooded back of the American Sergeant I met on gun pit duty one night at Nui Dat. I decided to go and visit him in Billings, Montana.***

Back in the room that night I woke in a panic in the middle of a nightmare. I was in a cold sweat and could smell smoke. I thought I was in Vietnam but then realised it wasn't a nightmare, it was real. The hotel across the road from mine was on fire. I raced to the window and watched people scramble for their lives down the fire escape ladders.

My journey continued by Greyhound bus from the Big Apple across to Chicago where I stayed for two days and then on the bus again via Minneapolis to Billings, Montana.

> ***After viewing the fall of Saigon and the end of the Vietnam War on TV I started to struggle again and slipped into a black hole of depression and loneliness. On the bus trip I ruminated for hours questioning about life, the Vietnam War, my sexual assault in the Army, the young lady that spat on me at Sydney airport, my sister's problems, and Scotty Wilson's death in Vietnam. I felt I was worthless with no future and thought again of disappearing into the freezing cold landscape to die peacefully.***

I arrived in Billings in the late evening after a thirty-hour trip and immediately booked into a hotel feeling exhausted. The next morning I went by taxi to the address on the scrap of paper. A young guy answered the door but looked puzzled when I said, "Looking for Ron Casey, mate. Does he live here?" He didn't seem to know Ron, so I returned to the taxi and was just about to move on when he came running out. "I know Ron Casey but not a Ron Caseymate!"

He was confused by my Aussie accent and adding 'mate' to Casey. Bob Feisthamel, nicknamed Feisty, had gone to school with Ron and knew where his mum lived. After paying the cab driver, I went inside with Feisty and he contacted Ron's mum. Ron was living in Helena, Montana. Later that evening I contacted him, and he instantly recognised my voice. (Must have been that Aussie accent again!)

This was the most defining time of my life till then. I believe that scrap of paper with Ron's address and meeting Feisty saved my life, because within that thirty seconds after leaving the house and getting into the taxi I had made up my mind, saying to myself, "STUFF IT, I am going to do myself in." Feisty rescued me from a deep lonely hole of depression.

In the end I stayed with Feisty for a week. He showed me all around the area including the site of the Battle of the Little Bighorn, also called Custer's Last Stand (June 25, 1876). Like me, Feisty was a Vietnam veteran but we never talked about the Vietnam War. Feisty had started skydiving and wanted me to go up with him and try it but the trouble was I couldn't get into the plane because of my PTSD condition. In the week I was with Feisty we spent a lot of time in the bars drinking and playing snooker, but he had found skydiving as a distraction from his problems, I guess from his Vietnam service. I'm still in contact with Feisty. He became a member the United States skydiving team and has done more than 8,400 jumps. Also, he has won 14 gold medals in 13 U.S. National Skydiving Championships and three gold and five silver medals in nine World Skydiving Championships, not to mention holding four world skydiving records.

It was a happy and emotional meet up with Ron when I finally arrived in Helena. Ron worked as the local postie and had married Sandy, an art teacher. For the next month I was spoilt with American hospitality, including a 'Welcome to Helena' party arranged for me, cross-country skiing and drives in the magnificent Montana countryside. For the first time since I returned from Vietnam, all my issues receded to the back of my mind. Even Ron didn't mention the war. He'd obviously moved on and was getting on with his life. I headed back to my sister's place in Portland for a couple weeks but found it depressing with the state of her marriage problems. I moved onto Seattle for a further two weeks where I stayed with my sister's friends and then back on the road again to Helena.

Ron and Sandy and their friends were the first people to really see that I was struggling with my life and helped me with my heavy drinking and ongoing avoidance of my problems. Their understanding and help were a timely reminder that I needed to get my act together.

Ron and Sandy were both into fitness and health which turned out a blessing for me. They could see I was struggling with life with the booze, so with their network of friends got me going again. The biggest hurdle was to get me out of the bars. They set out a plan for me. Every morning they got me up early and into a routine of exercise like bike rides or an early morning run. They introduced daily goals, like chopping and carting wood, gardening work, or cleaning and helping their friends with any odd jobs. They introduced me to cross country skiing and rock climbing. Every day was set up with some activity that would stimulate my brain and provide distraction from my problems and negative thoughts, increase my energy levels and above all provide motivation and a sense of achievement. I owe my life to Ron, Sandy and their friends of Helena, Montana.

It was a sad farewell when I finally departed and headed back to my sister's place for another month before farewelling her and her family.

On my return to Australia, I stopped off at Hawaii and did all the touristy things including a tour of Pearl Harbor.

I wanted to stay in America, didn't want to leave but my money had run out and six months leave from work was almost up. I had mixed feelings on the flight back to Australia. I began to wonder what the future held for me. For a short time, I had escaped the anger and mistrust of my own country. I felt that my countrymen might turn on me again and assumed other Vietnam veterans shared the same feelings. In America I simply felt accepted. I was determined to set immediate and long-term goals for myself. One of them was to save money, return to America and hopefully work in Canada. The other goal was to go back to night school and study for my Senior Certificate.

CHAPTER 14

BACK HOME – STUDY AND TRAINING

In mid-August 1975 I was back at work and enrolled in night school to complete my Senior certificate in Physics and Maths. I was off the booze and feeling better, but I was still having nightmares and anxiety attacks.

On my return to Brisbane I had trouble finding accommodation but eventually moved into a flat at Newmarket with a workmate, Jacky. After a while, my twin brother Don joined us. The flat was part of an old Queenslander home that had been turned into two flats. The flat next door was occupied by a middle-age couple and their young daughter about twelve years old. Sadly, I soon discovered the couple were alcoholics, binge drinking most days and nights, especially on weekends. The noise of banging bottles, breaking furniture, screaming arguments, and the most disturbing of all, sounds of vomiting echoed through our flat most of the time. Plus, we had to put up with the stench of cigarette fumes and a distinct rotten smell of sickness that lingered in the flat. The place pushed us to our limits, but we were lucky as we had only signed a three-month contract for the flat.

> ***I recognised for the first-time what alcohol can do to people lives. I felt relieved that I had managed to get off the booze especially with no cravings.***

The three of us then moved into a three-bedroom house in Ferny Hills in early December for six months. We settled into our new spacious surroundings quite well until the house next door was rented out to a large family of eight in early 1976. Our biggest problem with 'the family from hell' was they did not believe in rubbish bins and only used open rubbish bags on the back landing of the house. The stench of the rubbish attracted flies and with no fly screens in our house we were always battling flies, and this was not the only problem. When strong winds blew up, their rubbish would end up in our yard. Another big issue was their dog which always shat in our front and back yards. We made a few complaints to the council without success.

My **anger** and **frustrations** started to get out of control when Jacky went outside one evening to hang out clothes, accidently stepping on some dog turd and unknowingly treading it throughout the house. That took us hours to clean up. The next morning, I rang the council and they suggested we front the neighbour and complain but we had done this many times before and the complaints always fell on deaf ears so Jacky and I decided to get the message across by returning the dog turds in a way they would not forget. The family always had early dinner in the dining room with wide open windows near our back fence line. We thought that gave us the best opportunity to return the dog turds by shovel, heaving the turds through the open windows onto the dinner table. This we did, and hell erupted with screams and abuse. I yelled out, "Have that for tea, you bastards." The big lady screamed out, "You dirty, rotten, low-down bastards. I will get you both for that." Jacky shouted back, "You keep your fucking dog and rubbish in your back yard, you dirty, filthy bitch."

Soon the police arrived at our front doorstep with complaints from 'the family from hell'. We did not deny what we did and told our side of the story. In the end the police were understanding and sympathised with our situation and told the family to keep their dog chained up and keep their rubbish on their side of the fence. 'The family from hell' only lasted a further month in the house before the owners evicted them due to a fire in one of the bedrooms lit by one of the kids. It caused severe damage to the bedroom and added to the filthy condition of the house.

I noticed I had become extremely sensitive and critical of people's attitudes and behaviour, probably due to my time in the Army with its discipline and high standards of hygiene etc.

My focus was to complete my Senior certificate for Physics and Maths and to continue to work hard and save money, but my plans were set back when I lost all my possessions in a house fire in September 1976.

Our house lease expired and we moved from the Ferny Hills house into an old Queenslander in Gaythorne, but my twin brother Don did not last long and moved out because of the condition of the house. An electrical fault destroyed it a few months later. I lost all my furniture, clothes, books and personal belongings in the fire.

I was shattered but it could have been worse as the fire destroyed the house in the early hours of the morning with no one inside. I had three days off and had gone home to Caloundra and my workmate was on holiday in Bali. I wasn't insured so financially I was virtually broke. All I had left was the clothes I was wearing and the clothes I took home to be washed.

About the same time, I met a beautiful young lady by the name of Debbie Leabeater. After a whirlwind romance, we were engaged in November of the same year and married on the 5th March 1977, the day after my 29th birthday. Debbie 11 years younger than me had an upbringing like mine with no father. At the age of three, she had lost her father in tragic circumstances when he tried to break up a fight at a wedding and was stabbed and died in hospital shortly afterwards.

We went to the Barossa Valley in South Australia for our honeymoon and stayed in caravan parks. I wasn't too flush with money at the time, particularly having lost all my possessions in the fire. To make matters worse, a couple of weeks before the wedding, some lowlife stole Deb's engagement and friendship rings and my car roof rack, which I used for transporting my kayak, was stolen. I had to sell my kayak to help to fund the wedding and honeymoon.

On our return from the honeymoon, Deb and I moved into her mother's house to save money. We lived upstairs and her mother lived downstairs. It was not an ideal situation nor was it a good start to our marriage. It soon caused friction and numerous arguments.

> ***I was trying hard to save money and the combination of financial and emotional stress quickly made me aware of the short fuse of my temper. Within months, my marriage was on the rocks.***

I soon became restless again. I wanted to get out of Brisbane to diffuse the stress so we could move on and make some money. I decided to apply for two jobs, as a Technical Observer with the Bureau of Meteorology and for a Communication position with Foreign Affairs. I was successful with both applications but chose the Bureau job because of my fascination with the weather.

The Foreign Affairs job would require us to be living overseas on and off. Though appealing at first, it was not conducive to repairing my marriage and starting a family.

Deb and I moved to Melbourne to start the new job and hopefully refresh our marriage. I started my twelve months course in Melbourne on the 24th October 1977 at the Bureau of Meteorology Training School, Technical Observer's Course No 57. The course would help develop my knowledge and skills in an area in which I already had an interest.

There were fifteen of us on the course, all males from different backgrounds, including an ex-teacher, a pilot, an ambulance officer, an ex-Army Vietnam veteran, a champion angler and a few that worked in Meteorology like myself. On a tragic note, after one week of the course, one of the trainees drowned in the Goulburn River in northern Victoria on a weekend camping trip. We were all shattered.

> ***On the course with the added pressure of study and exams, I was experiencing anxiety attacks with body shakes and trembling especially when manually tracking weather balloons by radar and using a slide rule.***

My condition worsened as the year went on, so I went to a local doctor to get some tablets to calm me down, but he refused and instead sent me to a Psychiatrist. The Psychiatrist said I had severe War-like depression causing anxiety and wanted to put me into Heidelberg Repatriation Hospital. I refused to go into hospital, but in the end the Psychiatrist prescribed me some anxiety tablets which helped to calm me down. To continue with the tablets, I had to make monthly appointments to see him. I successfully completed my twelve-month course and was posted back to Queensland to Amberley Air Force Base along with another Vietnam veteran who was on my course. His name was Don McLeod, but his nickname was 'Grunt'. He was an Infantry soldier in Vietnam and his platoon was hit hard with a high rate of casualties. Like me he was having nightmares and not sleeping much. In Vietnam he had to put several of his mates into body bags. This was his recurring nightmare with their open eyes in death staring at him.

Before I headed back to Queensland the course had a graduation party in the backyard of an inner suburban house in Melbourne. Around forty attended including our instructors, girlfriends, wives and friends. It was a rip-roaring party enjoyed by all until one of our fellow trainee observers decided to let off a few big banger crackers under the Holden wagon in the driveway which the champion angler and his girlfriend had disappeared into.

This didn't go down well for me and 'Grunt'. My whole world was falling on top of me. It was Vietnam all over again. Only two of us hit the ground, 'Grunt' and me. Everyone laughed. My body was shaking all over before I returned to reality and realised what was going on. Poor 'Grunt' took off and clambered up a nearby tree, yelling: 'Where the fuck is the VC?' VC for Vietcong. Everyone thought he was yelling out: 'Where the fuck is the VB?' VB for Victoria Bitter beer. It must have been sight for sore eyes, me shaking on the ground, 'Grunt' up the tree and the champion angler and his girlfriend jumping out of the wagon half-naked.

'Grunt' and I were reliving our trauma through a flashback or panic attack. They are episodes of severe anxiety which can occur quite suddenly. We are born with a built-in alarm system to alert us to potentially life-threatening situations so we can either "fight or flee". They can last for a few minutes or sometimes longer. Common symptoms are a state of hyper-arousal, shortness of breath, trembling and shaking, feelings of unreality, dry mouth, muscle tension, unable to speak, pounding heart, nausea, sweating, losing control, a fear of dying and urge to flee.

CHAPTER 15

AMBERLEY

Relieved I had finally finished the course and done well, I took up my posting at Amberley Air Force Base from October 1978. I was working in a military environment, something I'd longed for when I first joined the Army in 1967, but at the same time I was a civilian. Deb and I shifted into a house in Ipswich owned by the Bureau of Meteorology. My fellow Vietnam vet, Don 'Grunt' lived at the Sergeants' Mess at the base.

'Grunt' and I would talk together at length about our Army and Vietnam experiences either in the mess or at work. Poor 'Grunt' couldn't relate to anyone else, even to the Air Force sergeants. When he wasn't on duty he would come into work and visit me. His conversations always focused on Vietnam. He had plenty of ghastly experiences, including killing and wounding a few VC and had seen lots of blood and guts. All this death and destruction weighed heavily on his mind, particularly when he had to pick up the bodies of his fallen mates and stuff them into body bags. I recall seeing body bags in choppers at various fire support bases. Just seeing the bags was traumatic enough and left a lasting effect on me. I couldn't imagine how it would feel to put your fallen mates into them. 'Grunt' lived for his annual leave, breaking up his leave every six months and heading to Thailand.

All this talk about Vietnam was causing havoc with my moods. My own experiences and fears which were tightly locked away were now being reopened. I became increasingly angry and aggressive and the people in the firing line were Debbie and my workmates. I became obsessive, picking up on tiny issues such as household cleanliness and neatness. Every little thing had to be in place, just like in the Army. I even took issue with Debbie and her healthy eating habits including all the low-fat foods she ate. My anger would bubble then explode as I thumped the walls shouting and upending chairs. I was living a nightmare within myself and Deb was one of the casualties.

Even at work I had an argument with my boss about cloud base heights. It was a minor issue but in hindsight it was more about my need to take control. He wanted me to change my forecast cloud base height to his. When I refused, he started shouting at me. I shouted back at him and told him to fuck off and leave me alone. My boss must have seen the anger boiling inside me and didn't say a word. Aware that 'Grunt' and I were both Vietnam veterans, he realised we had issues, that were not simply work-related.

Part of my job was to provide leave relief at Oakey Aviation Army Base. I had two long stints at Oakey, each of six weeks' duration and lived in the Sergeants' Mess which gave me a real feeling of what I'd escaped and left behind. I met a Vietnam veteran sergeant and I was horrified to learn that all he did was drink heavy booze. He hardly ate anything, just spent his days drinking at the bar including on weekends and holidays. He couldn't relate to anyone, just the booze.

> ***Deb threatened to leave me if I didn't do something about my anger and moods. I realised I had to do something to calm myself down as I couldn't handle it any longer. I went to a doctor to find out what I needed to do to reduce my anger and mood swings. He put me on tablets to calm my nerves and recommended that I should see a Psychiatrist. I didn't bother going to see the Psychiatrist as the tablets seemed to help.***

In November 1980, Deb and I left for six weeks holiday in America. On the second night after our arrival in San Francisco, a terrible nightmare woke me. My body shook in a cold sweat, and I gasped for breath as I struggled to find the light switch. The whole room seemed to be rocking and shaking. Deb, used to my nightmares woke briefly, but she promptly rolled back to sleep. When we arrived in the foyer that morning, the newspaper headline read, 'San Francisco Earthquake'. It was an earthquake of a magnitude 7.2 with the centre 65 kilometres away and damage relatively light. At least it explained to me the rocking and shaking room.

We had a busy six weeks, visiting my Vietnam mate, Ron and his wife Sandy. It was interesting to see how he continued to live his life. For Ron, Vietnam was in the past and he lived only for the future. Ron reminded me that I needed to do the same.

We also met up with another Vietnam veteran, David 'Bones' Bethka and his wife, Lanie in Kansas City. Bones a mate of Ron's had experienced horrendous combat in Vietnam. We got on the booze together and talked about Vietnam and politics in a way only Vietnam veterans can.

CHAPTER 16

LONGREACH

Time went quickly and before we knew it, we were back home packing and preparing for a move to Longreach in Central West Queensland in 1981. I was to fill a temporary promotion that offered an excellent opportunity to gain more experience, particularly with radar weather balloon flights.

Deb and I quickly settled into life at Longreach. During our stay I met another Vietnam veteran. He mentioned marching on Anzac Day and asked if I'd like to come along. I wasn't keen. In fact, I had avoided this very public event due to the miserable reaction of the general public and the thought of being a target for anti-war sentiment. I'd noticed people in the rural areas appeared more supportive of veterans than city people, so I decided I would march. The reality was no different and my expectations of a pride-filled march were destroyed. There were only about four Vietnam veterans marching including one who said he was a Vietnam veteran but wore no medals. He had plenty of booze in him and kept singing loudly, 'Onward Christian Soldiers Marching Off to War'.

> *I marched with feelings of inexplicable guilt and embarrassment. We were treated as a joke as people openly laughed at us. Our pride was given another kick as the old diggers were acknowledged and cheered. I had also served my country and experienced the horrors of war. The hypocrisy of it made my gut turn. I vowed never to march again.*

About two months into my new posting, I got word Don 'Grunt' McLeod had committed suicide in Thailand from a shotgun bullet to his head. He often said to me he would find peace in Thailand and he did. After I left Amberley, I guess he didn't have anyone to speak to, to ease his demons.

> *It took me a while to get over that tragic news.*
>
> *Guilt weighed me down heavily. I felt I had let down another mate, like I did with Robert 'Scotty' Wilson. I knew his issues was just like my own, but I kept asking myself did I do enough to help him. 'Grunt' liked reading and travelling and I encouraged him to keep saving and continue to travel overseas on holidays and even suggested he join a Book Club. Loneliness was his big issue. I was lonely when I first travelled to the USA in 1975. It is a dark place, like walking on a path without any directions. 'Grunt' only had one friend and that was me. Like me he feared people and did not trust anyone, but I was fortunate I found love and had a good family and friends. I know 'Grunt' had elderly parents, but he did not speak much about them. Unfortunately, there were no organisations available then to help veterans. The*

Vietnam Veterans Association of Australia (VVAA) was formed later, in 1979, to help Vietnam veterans with their health and their children's.

CHAPTER 17

IN THE RELIEF POOL

After 12 months in rural Longreach, it was a shock to be transferred back to Brisbane to the Relief pool in 1982. For the next two years I was posted to different offices around Queensland. I spent time working in Amberley, Longreach, Rockhampton, Cairns and the rest of the time at either Brisbane Airport or the Brisbane Forecast Centre.

The constantly shifting lifestyle suited me. Rockhampton was my preferred relief posting, and I enjoyed the work, particularly briefing pilots. I became friendly with several pilots at Rockhampton, including Alan Tricky, nicknamed 'Tricky Dicky', who grew up in Caloundra. Tricky offered me a return flight to Brisbane on the nightly freight run, I accepted. Loaded with general cargo, the Cessna type 402 had the call sign DIL. The only way to get to the cockpit was to crawl over the boxes and satchel bags. This freaked me out, and I had flashbacks of the pit hole in Vietnam. Somehow, I managed to crawl through the small gap between the cargo and ceiling to the cockpit seat.

I asked Tricky, "In an emergency, how do you get out of this flying box? I reckon we'd be in a lot of shit if we crashed."

He just laughed, "You'd have to kick your way out through the cockpit, or this might help." Tricky handed me a tomahawk from behind his seat.

The trip down to Brisbane was perfect with clear skies.

I was still experiencing waves of anxiety.

On the return trip to Rockhampton at around 3am, we climbed to a cruising altitude. Tricky put the heater on to warm us up and flicked the plane onto auto pilot. The groaning of the engine and the warmth from the heater quickly put us both to sleep. It must have been at least 15 minutes before I woke in the middle of a nightmare. Tricky jumped awake too. He noticed the Cessna had dropped 1500 metres.

"Shit, I'll have to report this problem," he said.

Tragically a few days later, Cessna 402 call sign DIL crashed into a mountain range in Central Queensland killing a budding Rockhampton pilot.

I never heard the official cause of the tragic accident, but I always wondered if it was the same problem we'd experienced a few days earlier with the altitude lock.

In mid-September 1983, I completed my time in Rockhampton and returned to work at Brisbane Airport for a month before starting a month's leave. This was planned just in time for the birth of our first child. Our daughter, Michelle Ann, was born on 17th October 1983.

Shortly afterwards, I was posted to Cairns on a temporary relief for five months. It took us three full days to get there in hot humid conditions and with no air-conditioner in the car, I felt sorry for our four weeks old baby, Michelle, in her bassinette on the back seat. We booked into a self-contained two-bedroom holiday unit not far from the hospital on the Esplanade. The only drawbacks with the unit were the lack of air-conditioning and no screens on the windows.

We settled well into our new surroundings until in January, I came down with Dengue fever which is a mosquito-borne tropical disease caused by the dengue virus. I felt like dying with a high fever, severe headaches, vomiting, agonizing pain in my joints, skin rash, fatigue and **depression**. I was in bed for four weeks virtually. All up I had a month off work, but it took me a further month to fully recover and get my strength back.

One morning at 4am during my illness, Debbie was sitting on the couch breast feeding Michelle in the dark. Facing the open kitchen window she noticed a shadowy figure trying to get through it. She screamed out "Hey," and I quickly jumped out of bed and saw the would-be thief scrambling back out. I chased the surprised intruder down the street but weak as I was, soon lost him in the dark.

In March 1984, Deb noticed a lump growing on baby Michelle's toe. Both of us were concerned when the cyst continued to grow. A specialist at Cairns Hospital told us it was a rare growth called infantile digital fibroma and recommended an operation to remove the growth and half her toe. The cyst was about eight millimetres, bigger than a pea and bright red.

I've always reckoned it was a legacy of my exposure to Agent Orange in Vietnam. A lot of Vietnam veterans including me had been subjected to the deadly foliage spray and many of our children present with disfigurement, health problems or both.

In late April we returned to Brisbane and Michelle was admitted to the Royal Brisbane Hospital where the growth was removed.

The growth never returned.

CHAPTER 18

CHARLEVILLE

In August 1984 I took a new job at Charleville in outback south-west Queensland. I enjoyed the rural location and my new job enormously. Unfortunately, I soon found out that it wasn't as perfect as I had anticipated as I discovered that my boss didn't like me. Worse still, he lived next door to us. He accused me of different things such as leaving work early which I never did and doing wheelies outside the Met building after heavy rain, churning up the mud.

He called the police and wanted me arrested. "There's the guilty person," the boss said pointing his finger at me. "He's the one who has been doing all the wheelies outside this building for months. Look at his wheels. They're full of red mud, and he was the only person on duty this morning."

The copper replied to the boss after checking my wheels and the boss's wheels. "That's no evidence whatsoever. You've got as much mud on your wheels. Even my wheels are the same."

The wheelies persisted, particularly after rainy days, while the grumbles continued from the boss. In the end the Met building cleaner told me privately, he was the phantom wheelie-maker to shit stir the boss.

The situation grew worse when our little boy, David William, was born on the 13th August 1985 and I was on special leave from work to look after Michelle. The boss continued to harass me regarding the length of time I was entitled to and when I would be back at work.

I was upset and reported the incident to our Senior Admin Officer in Brisbane who told me not to worry and that special leave was my entitlement.

In the early stage of Deb's pregnancy, she had lost a great deal of blood (miscarriage), so it was a surprise to us all to find that she was still pregnant. I will always wonder whether, once again, this had something to do with Agent Orange in Vietnam.

In late 1986, the Bureau decided to have a bulk promotion exercise for Meteorology Observer Grade 2 positions. I applied for three positions, including the position in which I was acting at Charleville. I was rated above average from all my former bosses but below average by my current boss. I was stunned and pissed off. I wrote at the bottom of the report sheet that I disagreed with the report, but in the end, I could do nothing about it. I had a go at my boss, but it was like speaking to a brick wall.

With all the hassle of the promotion exercise, I couldn't sleep and couldn't eat, which caused my body to run down. I developed a large boil on my backside and subsequently developed a fever. Feeling decidedly unwell, I visited our local doctor, who lanced the boil with a scalpel and drained it.

It was very painful and unpleasant but surprising how quickly it healed after he gave me antibiotics.

In early 1987, the list of successful applicants for promotion to Grade 2 positions was published in the Commonwealth Public Gazette. Unfortunately, my name was not on the list. I rang the Regional boss in Brisbane who said I'd just missed out because of my boss' report. I was consumed with **anger**. Determined that justice would prevail, I decided to lodge an appeal with the Chairman of the Promotions Appeal Committee against all the successful applicants. This was a difficult process as I had to prove to the Committee that I was a better officer at my job, in knowledge and ability, as well as in attitude, than the successful applicants. I also had to prove that the Selection Committee got it wrong.

My appeal was held in late April 1987 by phone link to Brisbane and the interview lasted an hour. In the end, the three-person committee on the Appeals Panel found the Selection Committee had failed to recognise my experience, and that a personality clash with my boss had affected my rating.

I was promoted to Grade 2, replacing the last officer on the promotion list. I felt a huge relief that justice had finally prevailed. My boss did not utter a word to me. I knew he hated my guts. It was mutual. I decided to look for the first opportunity to get out of Charleville.

On an afternoon shift in late 1987, I experienced a severe bout of **anxiety** when one of the Flight Service Officers fired a shotgun with a blank to scare off birds in the area to prevent aircraft suffering bird strike. I was taking temperatures from our Stevenson screen in the enclosure at the time, and it scared the living daylights out of me. It was like reliving Vietnam. I hit the ground and it took about thirty seconds before I could compose myself. The Flight Service Officer thought it was a great joke as I didn't let on to him that I was a Vietnam veteran.

The final knockout blow with the boss came when I fronted him about an incident that happened a couple of days before the Bicentenary celebrations on 26th January 1988 when he showed three local councillors through the office. I suggested I release the balloon ten minutes early so they could watch the release and radar tracking.

The boss ridiculed me on the spot. "You know the rules, Morgan. You do not, I repeat do not, release the balloon before time, only between ten minutes to twenty past the hour. Do you hear me, Morgan?"

I felt embarrassed and belittled and wanted to crawl under the desk. I stood speechless in shock and remained in the same spot until the entourage had left the building. I couldn't sleep and fumed about the incident all night as hatred and aggression built within me. I felt there was no excuse for his outburst, particularly in front of strangers.

On the day of the Bicentenary celebration, I completed my shift at 1.00 pm and the boss took over. I took my family down to the showgrounds to celebrate the special day. At around 3.00 pm, I couldn't believe my eyes when I saw my boss at the showgrounds selling hamburgers and celebrating. So much for office protocol. When he came to work the next afternoon to take over the shift, I was waiting for him. I'd been stewing over the earlier incident and this was the final blow. I couldn't wait to confront him.

Eyeballing him I angrily said, "I don't like the way you had a go at me a few days back in front of strangers. If you have something to say to me, tell me behind closed doors. You say you follow the rules and never take short cuts with your work."

The boss looked nervous and started breathing heavy. "Yes, and I expect my staff to follow rules," he retorted.

"Don't tell me that bullshit, you filthy liar. I saw you at the celebration yesterday when you were supposed to be at work. You follow the rules, but you cut short your balloon flight and made up your hourly weather reports, you hypocritical bastard."

It was the first time in my life I had felt like smashing someone, smashing his bloody face in. My boss must have seen the anger in my eyes because he stepped back and quickly left the room. Had he been a little closer, I have no doubt I would have been on an assault charge. We never spoke again, and from then on, he always went out of his way to avoid me.

CHAPTER 19

GLADSTONE

In late February 1988, I received the good news that I was to be transferred to a permanent position at the Gladstone office. My new boss was supportive and sincere towards his staff and treated everyone equally. We settled into the Gladstone lifestyle routine with the enjoyment of my new job and family activities.

It was a welcome change.

I became involved in soccer, coaching my son, David's team. Through soccer I met another Vietnam veteran and he talked me into joining the local Vietnam Veteran's Association (VVAA). Once a month we would meet for a barbeque.

For the first time since Vietnam, I felt comfortable talking to strangers on different subjects and realised that Vietnam had taken its toll on us veterans. There were guys just like me, who were struggling with common issues. It was a real eye-opener and made me realise that I wasn't the only one alone and harbouring problems. I think we had simply accepted the fact that people didn't want to hear about our experiences, our war, and had shut down communications.

At one of the monthly meetings, I was voted in as a Welfare Officer. This position involved me visiting a fellow Vietnam veteran who had served as a gunner on choppers. He'd seen so many disturbing things during his service and after 20 years he continued to have difficulty dealing with his experiences. In response to his struggle with life, he went on booze binges, hit his wife and kids, and even attempted suicide.

For someone who wasn't great at managing my own demons, I wasn't sure exactly what I would be able to do to help someone so burdened with life.

My job was to talk to him and offer any assistance that VVAA could provide. He found it easy to relate to me and would sometimes come over to my house for a chat. Sadly, he tried suicide again and ended up in hospital where I visited him. Helping him wasn't helping me, as my **nightmares and anxiety** attacks increased. Of course, putting two people who were equally screwed up over Vietnam together just wasn't going to work.

After three weeks I relinquished the position, realising that every time I met my fellow veteran, it was like looking into a mirror, his problems reflecting mine.

In October 1990, Deb, Michelle, David and I went for a holiday in America for six weeks. We visited Disneyland and Universal

Studios. We also caught up with my Vietnam mates and their families. It was good to see Dave 'Bones' Bethka and his wife, Lanie now living outside Phoenix, Arizona and Ron and Sandy Casey and their two girls, still living in Helena, Montana.

> ***I felt at home. Their hospitality was overwhelming, and I felt more relaxed in America than in my real home in Australia. In Australia I still hold bad memories from when I returned home from Vietnam like being verbally abused and spat on. In America, I never experienced anything like that, only good memories.***

On the 20th February 1992 I was promoted to Officer in Charge of the Gladstone Meteorology Office. I was now responsible for running the station. It entailed supervising all staff members and representing the Bureau on the Gladstone District Disaster Control Group as well as acting as a Port Meteorological Agent servicing five vessels in Gladstone Port.

After one early shift, I went home to get some sleep, a standard routine for me. I woke when I heard screams at the front door. It was our next-door neighbour holding her two-year-old grandson, Troy. Alison regularly babysat little Troy. I took one look at the toddler and could see right away that this was a desperate situation. His face was pale blue and he was frothing at the mouth. Alison was beside herself. Apparently Troy had drunk mineral turpentine from a milk bottle while she had been painting the house. Under pressure I told Alison who was in a state of panic to get into the back seat of my car which was parked in the driveway. I drove to the Ambulance Centre a kilometre away and broke all traffic rules including going through a red light. On entry to the Centre I grabbed the little boy from Alison and handed him to a startled Ambulance Officer. Straight away they were in a speeding ambulance to the Gladstone Hospital. An ambulance officer later told me I had made the right decision to drive to the Centre instead of the Hospital to save crucial time in a dire situation. That night Alison and Troy's parents came to thank me for my quick actions in saving Troy's life.

> ***I wonder whether I would have taken the same action and had a clear mind in a crisis without my Army training or Vietnam experience. However, it disturbed me that I felt no emotion whatsoever, just a numb feeling.***

On the evening of the 15th March 1992, the Regional Director of Queensland Bureau of Meteorology rang me at home and asked me to man the weather radar after 11.00pm. The weather station was normally unmanned between 11.00pm and 2.30am. Cyclone Fran, a Category 2 cyclone, was situated just off the coast near Heron Island. I left home just before 11.00pm to drive up the hill. Never will I again venture outside in cyclonic winds, as I fought the elements of nature. With tree branches strewn all over the road, strong gale force winds and blinding rain limited my visibility as I drove up Radar hill. Usually, the drive to the Met office from my place takes 5 minutes. This hazardous trip took me 15 minutes. Once I got to the safety of the Met office, my duties were to take pictures of Cyclone Fran on the radar and send them to the Cyclone Centre in Brisbane by fax machine. Around midnight I was joined by the OIC of Gladstone police, the head of SES and the big boss from Gladstone Alumina Plant to monitor the movement of Cyclone Fran.

This was one of the most stressful moments I have experienced, especially being forced to leave my family to face the Cyclone by themselves. My anxiety levels were high, the worst I have felt since my Vietnam days but once I started my commute to the Met station, I again had a clear mind in a crisis due to my Army training. Someone had to do it as there was no other way of finding the correct location of the cyclone. So I went with a strong sense of duty to the local community and the adrenaline rush took over.

Cyclone Fran made landfall on the Queensland coast near the Town of 1770 during March 16th. Eventually the severe Tropical Cyclone turned towards the southeast and headed back out to sea.

On the 26th August 1992, my dear Mum passed away in the Gladstone Hospital. She suffered a severe stroke in early 1991 so Debbie and I decided to take care of her for nine months until we got her into Alchera Park Nursing home just outside Gladstone. She died from an infection that spread from the pins that supported her broken hip, caused when she had stumbled on Council road works in Caloundra during my junior year at High School. Before her passing, a surgeon had operated to remove the pins in the infected area. She was frail and passed away two weeks after the operation.

Mum was an amazing lady, raising four children by herself, our dad having died before my twin brother and I were born. I will miss her forever.

In 1992, the Bureau advised all the staff at Gladstone Met that the station would close in early 1993. On 7th April 1993,

Gladstone Met Station launched its last weather balloon and the following day completed its last weather observation ending 35 years of operations. I closed the doors for the last time on 14th June 1993.

CHAPTER 20

WORKING IN ROCKHAMPTON BUT LIVING IN YEPPOON

In late June I was redeployed to Rockhampton Office at the airport in charge of the Observer section.

In the meantime, we bought a house in Yeppoon, 40 minutes from Rockhampton. Sport played an important part in my life during my time at Rockhampton. In fact, it became an obsession. It provided another outlet.

I was trying my best to get away from thoughts of Vietnam, although my nightmares and anxiety attacks were increasing.

On the 20th January 1994 Cyclone Rewa came within 100km of the coast and caused flash flooding around Brisbane which resulted in four deaths. Also, two men from a fishing trawler were rescued by Army helicopter as their vessel sank off the coast near

Yeppoon. At the time there was a lot of pressure at work from the media and the public especially from incoming telephone calls wanting the position of cyclone Rewa. I came on duty at 4.30 pm for the 12-hour shift. When I arrived, the media, WIN-TV, was doing live updates for TV with the boss.

The boss finished work at 6.00pm as did the TV mob, leaving their cameras, erected lights and gear in the Office. At the time I thought it was odd, but I was shocked and surprised when they turned up at 8.00pm for live updates as my boss failed to mention it to me. The reporter and TV cameraman said they had permission from my boss, so I had no alternative but to let them into the office.

For the next six hours it was total chaos, as the young lady reporter and cameraman took over the whole office. I could hardly move in the operation area of my workplace with all their gear and live TV updates. I was under enough pressure as it was, with my normal work load, releasing a weather balloon at 9.15 pm, tracking it by radar, coding and sending out the Upper Winds by telex, answering nonstop incoming telephone calls, sending out Special Aerodrome Meteorological reports every half hour and three hourly Synoptic Observations.

The situation was magnified more as they continued to move in and out of my operation area using our telephone lines for technical details to their TV station. My final boiling point or breaking point came when I discovered the lady reporter had ripped off the latest Cyclone Warning from the telex printer without my knowledge and permission and was doing a live broadcast update on camera.

I had been waiting patiently a good ten minutes for the

warning to come off the printer so I could telephone different Emergency Organizations.

I exploded in an explicit way, "You do NOT touch anything in this office, especially incoming latest Cyclone Warnings without my permission and knowledge. As far as I am concerned that's it. You both can get out of here and stop bloody interfering with my workplace."

The lady reporter kept on arguing, "We have responsibilities too."

I answered. "Maybe so, but you do not take anything off the telex, or touch anything without permission. How would you like me to go and touch your gear and camera? Oh no that's different."

They left about 1.30am leaving their gear. I felt like chucking it out with them. After I got home that morning I couldn't sleep.

> ***I started ruminating. I was repetitively going over the problem in my mind. Rumination commonly occurs with anxiety and depression.***

I decided to type a letter to the Regional Director of Qld, stating the chaotic situation that occurred that night at work should not be repeated. My main grumble was that the Officer-In-Charge (OIC) failed to inform me about the media coming in to do live updates on the cyclone and his lack of communication. Also, I stated he failed to recognise requirements or orders from the Cyclone Directory. In the Cyclone Directory it reads, 'No media allowed in the operation area that disturbs the operations.' I stated the TV crew constantly restricted my movement within my workplace plus they interfered by taking a cyclone warning from the printer without my knowledge and permission.

The next day I fronted the OIC straight away with my concerns. He didn't seem too interested at first, but that changed when I produced the letter for the Regional Director. I said to the boss, "I want you to read this letter, before I forward it onto the Regional Director. It is a complaint about you and the TV crew."

After he finished reading the letter, he looked nervous and started apologizing to me for the lack of communications on his behalf, plus the pressure I was put under from the media.

He then asked me to withdraw the letter of complaint to the Regional Director. "I'm sorry, Dave." And he continued. "It is not worth it. We both would be put under extreme pressure, if you go ahead with this letter. Let's keep our problems within the office. I certainly will take heed of my faults."

For me it was enough. I didn't want to cause any strife within the office, plus I wanted a healthy working relationship with my boss. I didn't want it to become like Charleville all over again. I decided to bite my tongue and move on with life.

From then onwards all the blame seemed to centre on the WIN-TV crew. The media apologized and the fallout began with the WIN-TV producer sacked and the lady reporter transferred to another WIN-TV station.

I noticed the boss gave me more respect and lifted his communication skills dramatically.

In May 1995 I went to Victoria for three weeks to attend a combined training course. It included lectures on basic meteorology, presentation skills, media skills, client relations, customer service, behaviour, leadership and team performance roles. When I returned from the course, I distributed numerous Meteorological Information kits to libraries, schools and shire councils around the district. All this work combined with my normal shift work and sporting commitments began taking a toll on me. I knew something had to give, particularly when I became increasingly short-tempered, frustrated and impatient.

The first signs came when a parent had a go at me while I was trying to organise a scratch match with a shortage of players at an Under Seventeen Australian Rules match in Yeppoon.

It happened when a smart-arse player in our team had a go at me in the dressing room in front of parents and supporters. "Why don't you shut your fucking big mouth, piss off and get out of here," he yelled at me.

I instantly saw red. "Don't you ever talk to me in that manner." I retorted. "Either show some respect, smart arse or you don't play."

I was in the middle of the heated argument when a loudmouth parent abused the shit out of me because of my attitude. "I don't like your attitude. You shouldn't talk to the boys like that." He said.

I saw red again. "Okay mate, you have a go at me, but in the end I don't see you lifting a finger by giving up your spare time, travelling to meetings during the week, or putting your hand in your pockets for fuel or manning scoreboards, being a timekeeper, umpiring and organising games. Here's the clipboard, mate. You are now Junior Vice President. I quit." The bloke was stunned as I walked out and went home.

The fight over a lack of respect or appreciation for what I was doing had stirred up the same confused feelings I had when I returned from Vietnam.

The Club apologised to me and forced the 16-year-old kid to apologise, however my love for junior sport died that day. It was the same with soccer. I found most parents didn't appreciate or care two hoots and only a handful turned up to help. They only cared for their little Johnny being babysat on Saturday mornings and for two hours training one night a week.

My sporting commitments during winter: Every Saturday I coached my junior soccer team for Yeppoon United Soccer Club and on Sunday I was the Junior Vice President for the Yeppoon Australian Rules Football Club. If I was rostered on day shift for weekends at work, I would have to swap shifts with my fellow shift workers to attend matches.

My **nightmares** and **anxiety** attacks increased. In the mornings, my pillows were soaking wet with sweat after I had suffered unescapable nightmares. Sometimes I was too scared to sleep, which left me even more tired. With 12-hour shifts at work, I became a walking zombie. I discovered that my body clock slowed down between the hours of 4.00 am and 6.00 am, particularly before sunrise, and I often found myself nodding off at work or on the long trip home to Yeppoon after I finished work in the early mornings.

On one freezing morning at 4.30 am going home after a twelve-hour shift on a straight stretch of road, with the heater on and the windows up, I simply fell asleep. I thought I was home in bed in a deep sleep, dreaming of this flashing bright light coming towards me. I must have only nodded off for three or four seconds, but it was just enough for my vehicle to cross to the wrong side of the road. To this day, I don't know what woke me, but I woke with a jerk and quickly realised I was not in bed, I was in my car with another vehicle flashing their lights coming towards me.

> *It scared the living daylights out of me but I knew I had to do something about my fear of sleep and my increasing exhaustion.*

The Singapore Army and Air Force and the Australian Defence Force held a combined military exercise in late October and November every year. The whole of Rockhampton airport was abuzz with military aircraft flying in and out including the Singapore Air Force choppers which parked about 50 metres from our Met office. There were about ten choppers coming and going all hours of the day and night over the four-week exercise period. The sounds of the choppers began to give me flashbacks from Vietnam. By the time the exercise finished, I was a nervous wreck. I'd had enough of everything in general and in a reasonably extreme decision I decided to apply for a remote posting at Giles Weather Station in the Gibson Desert, situated south-west of Alice Springs, for six months.

> *I just wanted to get away from the entire world. I discovered it was the little things that affected my equilibrium. My ability to function, my perception of everyday life was tainted by what I'd been through.*

CHAPTER 21

IN THE DESERT AT GILES

The Giles station is situated about 750 kms west-southwest of Alice Springs, just over the West Australian border, on the edge of the Gibson Desert and south of the Rawlinson Range. The Weather Station was established in 1956 by the Weapons Research Establishment, a division of the Department of Defence. The purpose of the station was to provide weather data for the UK atomic weapons tests at Emu Plains and Maralinga. It was also used to support the Rocket testing program at Woomera. Giles weather station was transferred from the Dept of Defence to the Bureau of Meteorology in 1972. I was successful in my application for the OIC position at Giles for six months and took up the position in early March 1998.

> *It was not an easy decision to leave my family, but I felt my health was in a downward spin. I was suffering from a lot of anxiety attacks and mental blocks at Rocky, and with shift work, I felt all these issues were putting my family under*

enormous pressure which they could do without. I didn't want to uproot my family as Michelle and David were in their important years of secondary school, so I decided six months posting away from home probably would be the best way to solve all these issues.

Most of my friends question why I was leaving my family. One lady commented "I know if it was my husband, I'd kick him out of the door for good." I honestly couldn't be bothered arguing and telling them the real reason was my struggle with anxiety and depression.

In the late afternoon on the 4th March, my birthday, I went up to Water Park Creek outside Yeppoon to say goodbye to David at his school camp. It was hard for me to say goodbye. I felt like a real bastard of a father thinking I'll not be seeing or supporting my son for the next six months. I was questioning myself, why am I doing this? The next day, 5th March, I was full of emotion when I said goodbye to Deb and Michelle at Rockhampton Airport. I flew to Melbourne to do an Electrolyser course (machine making hydrogen gas).

On the 8th March I caught a flight to Adelaide where I had briefings at the Adelaide Regional Office with the Regional bosses regarding my duties and responsibilities as OIC of Giles. On the 11th March I flew by Qantas flight to Alice Springs where I met up with my four ingoing crew members (three Met Technical Observers and one General Hand/Mechanic). We then caught a Ngaanyatjarra Air flight, a twin-engine plane to Giles. We landed at Giles dirt airstrip at around mid-afternoon nearby the Weather station. All up the trip took about three hours, including a fuel stop at Yulura.

There was no wasting time for the changeover, as all the new ingoing crew members had to work and familiarize with their duties that evening. It wasn't easy for me as I had to be briefed not only on my normal work duties but also with OIC duties ordering food stores plus the whole running of the station. The outgoing OIC took me into Warrakurna, an aborigine community just down the road from Giles, to meet the aborigine elders plus the white administrators. Giles Weather Station is a modern fully equipped station which carries out a full range of Meteorological observations, including upper atmosphere observations using balloon flights and radar tracking. It is the only staffed weather station in an area of about 2.5 million square kilometres. It is a key station for climate measurement and forecasting purposes over much of Australia, especially its location, as it is near the core of the subtropical jet stream. That evening we also had a big farewell dinner celebration for the outgoing crew. The old crew members left Giles the next morning by Ngaanyatjarra Air. The pilot had stayed at Giles overnight for the changeover period.

For the first few weeks we had problems with the Electrolyzer machine and communications equipment but after contacting the Meteorology technician in Alice Springs we soon sorted out the communications. The Electrolyzer was a bigger problem as someone accidentally put bore water instead of demineralized water into the machine. The Met technician had to come from Alice Springs to fix the problem. Even the weather gods weren't kind to us when we recorded 38.8 mm from thunderstorms and rain. This caused roads to be closed and thick mud everywhere. The good thing about the rain was it made the Giles area look alive with the flora and vegetation, especially the different desert flowers blooming to life with beautiful colours.

At the end of March I had my first trip out of Giles. Our mechanic and I travelled to Docker River to pick up our monthly food supply. Docker River is about 100 kms from Giles just over the Northern Territory border. The trip along the muddy road by Land Rover took us about two hours. Our monthly supplies were transported from Alice Springs to Docker River store by semi-trailer at the end of each month. It was my duty as OIC to put a food order in by fax to a supplier in Alice Springs at the end of each month.

After a couple of hours loading the Land Rover and checking the food order, we drove back to Giles with the road full of mud holes. I noticed several old ruined cars or car bodies abandoned on the side of the road. I soon discovered the aborigines would drive their cars to the very end and then would dump them on the side of the road. Over time other aborigines would come along in their old cars to retrieve any good spare parts. Eventually with time only the rusting car body remained.

Life at Giles was going smoothly for me until mid-April when our bore water pump broke down which meant no water for our showers and toilets. Lucky for us, Hans, our General Service Hand/Mechanic, had lifted a bore before. It would have taken a couple of weeks for someone to come in and fix it, so for the next three days it was all hard sweaty and dirty work for Hans and me as we set up a chain pulley and lifted the rods out with clamps. We soon discovered that some of the buckets on the rods had broken away causing the problem.

The meaning of remoteness and isolation was soon realised as we couldn't go down the road to an industrial workshop and buy buckets.

Hans and I had to go back to our workshop and make some new buckets and clamps, then came the arduous job of fixing the newly made buckets to the rods and dropping the rods down the bore hole with the clamps using the chain pulley set up.

I realised how much responsibility I had in running the Station.

At the end of April, I got a phone call from the Bureau of Meteorology Chief Administrator Officer in Adelaide regarding the Wongai hut. When we first arrived at Giles, all the incoming crew members including myself had to pay $500 to get into the business of the Wongai hut and the tourist souvenirs. The Wongai hut was situated about 15 metres just outside our main mess/lounge building and catered for the aborigines' needs after the nearby Roadhouse closed daily at 6pm. We provided sandwiches, boiled eggs, cordial drinks, chocolates, lollies, potato chips and cigarettes. The person who had the day off would look after the Wongai hut, serving and making sandwiches and cordial.

The Wongai hut kept us all busy. To me it was a pain in the backside, as it put more pressure and anxiety onto me especially when I was trying to run a Weather Station. It was full on. I found it very frustrating and annoying, when I had to get up from my lounge chair while watching TV or at night when I was awakened by a honking car sound, requiring me to serve in the Wongai hut. On average we would serve about thirty customers a night. It was especially busy on pension days and when local football carnivals were held.

The investigation of the Wongai hut came about when one smart aleck clerk in Adelaide office discovered the cost of my food order was less than previous crew food orders by a big amount. He rang me a few times questioning my food order. “Are you blokes eating out there?” or “Are you blokes on a diet?” or “Don’t you blokes like bread and cordial”. After a few phone calls, he twigged that something fishy was going on so reported it to the Chief Administrator Officer. They soon discovered the previous Giles crew, had rorted the system by including the cost of bread, sandwich meat, cordial, eggs and other food items for the Wongai hut in the main food order account. I ordered separately from our main food order and charged on a separate account. The order was delivered to Docker River at the same time as our own main food order.

The Bureau was pretty pissed off and threatened to close the Wongai hut. I soon discovered this was the beginning of the long saga regarding the hut.

They also looked at the souvenirs that we were selling to the tourists calling in at Giles. The tourists could buy hat badges, key rings, spoons and postcards. A company somewhere in South Australia produced the souvenirs for us. The souvenirs were popular with the on-going tourists and we didn’t have any trouble selling them.

Nothing resulted from the investigation. I think the Bureau's main concern was if selling these souvenir items was interfering with our work duties.

In early June the Wongai hut saga was back on the agenda again for me. I had a phone call from the South Australia Regional Director stating that the Director of Meteorology in Melbourne had ordered the closure of the Wongai hut immediately. Disturbing issues had been brought to the Director's attention from one of the nurses at Warakurna complaining that the Met staff at Giles were using discarded or throw-away unhygienic plastic drink bottles for reuse for cordial drinks at the canteen hut. The nurse was concerned this was a health hazard to the aborigines. I didn't deny to the Regional Director that we were using throw-away plastic drink bottles, in fact I stated this procedure had been going on now for a few years. The cleaning of the plastic drink bottles was a rigorous sterilization procedure which usually would take a couple of days to complete. This procedure in hot boiling water with a bottle brush and detergent was repeated at least half a dozen times. As far as I know no aborigines had fallen ill in the years selling the cordial in plastic bottles at the hut. Another issue fronting the Director in Melbourne was from a disgruntled Met Observer who was kicked out of Giles previously. He wrote a letter to the Director or someone high up threatening to write a letter to the Australia Tax Office with regards to the illegal running of the hut canteen.

This apparently sent shivers up the big bosses of Meteorology in Melbourne. The next day I ordered my crew to close the Wongai hut. Later in the day the aborigines from Warakurna came rolling up to buy cordial, sandwiches, chocolates, cigarettes, etc at the hut but we had to tell them the bad news that the Wongai hut was closed for good by order from the big boss. The aborigines looked lost, confused, and angry and didn't seem to know what was going on. The next day the white administrator from the community fronted me asking what the hell was going on and said that he had a near riot on his hands from upset, angry aborigines with the closure of the Wongai Hut. I immediately contacted the Regional Director in Adelaide and the Director in Melbourne. Within days, a phone call came from the Regional Director telling me to reopen the hut canteen. The Bureau was negotiating with the Warakurna community for the canteen to be kept open until they could find another alternative means. Obviously, the Bureau wasn't expecting such a backlash from the Warakurna community with regards the closure of the Wongai hut. I heard later a petition was sent to the Bureau from the community.

The saga came to an end on Friday the 4th September when we finally closed the Wongai hut. The Warakurna community had negotiated with the roadhouse and the local store to extend their hours especially on weekends. We had instructions from the Bureau to give the Wongai hut to the community. On the Saturday the 5th the Wongai hut was transported by truck to the Warakurna football field.

> ***For me it was big relief to rid of this ongoing saga. The five of us made a profit of about one and half thousand dollars each.***

Wongai hut wasn't the only problem or challenge I had to face while at Giles. I soon discovered one of the Met Technical

Observers was a big problem to us all. It all started on a Sunday in early May. I had been on the earlier day shift and was relaxing, watching the footy on TV in the lounge room. The next thing I knew the front door burst opened and in walked Paul (Met Observer) with twenty tourists following behind him. I was dumbfounded when he went to the TV and turned the footy off and put on a video tape on four wheel-driving.

> ***My reaction? I was speechless and shocked at what was happening with all the strangers looking at me.***

The lounge and the Mess area were a no-go zone area, a private area for staff only, unless you are an invited guest.

In shock, I yelled out to Paul, "What are you doing? I'm watching footy."

Paul replied "Blow your footy. We want to watch a 4WD video. These tourists belong to a 4-Wheel Drive club."

I got up from my seat and saw red with **anger**. I yelled, "This is not on. This is a private area for staff only and you know the rules."

Paul replied, "Oh shut up. See, my friends, what I have to put up with from this boss of mine."

> ***I could see the strangers looking at me with a look of bemusement or embarrassment on their faces. I decided to leave the lounge room. I felt embarrassed, angry and in some ways, belittled. My mind flashbacked to the young lady who spat on me at Sydney Airport when I returned home from Vietnam and the incident with my OIC at Charleville when he belittled me in front of local councillors. I thought it was best to get out as the situation could have become nasty***

and out of control with my anger as I was beginning to lose control of my emotions.

Later in the day after the tourists had gone, I fronted Paul in my office and there was an exchange of heated words. He reckoned I was quite rude to the tourists. I pointed out the facts to him, that I would not tolerate his behaviour and I would be reporting him to the Regional Director of South Australia. As far as I was concerned, I wanted him out of Giles. I wasn't the only one who had issues with him. Other crew members were arguing with him. I rang the Regional Director (RD) about the incident. He was in total agreement with me and advised me to get rid of him and he would replace him with someone else for the remaining 4 months.

The RD told me he would give me a couple days to think about it. After two days I rang the RD with my decision. I decided to keep Paul at Giles. My thinking was if I got rid of him from Giles, the Bureau might think I couldn't handle difficult personnel or pressure situations. It would go onto my record and go against me in future promotions. The RD came back to me bluntly. "OK, don't call me in a month's time and say you can't handle him. You've made your decision and had your chance."

I had a feeling deep down I had made a big mistake and there would be troubled times ahead for me.

I only got a short break of peace before my mental suffering started again with arguments, fights and mounting tension between Paul and the other crew members. Once again it started with Paul. This time over lamb shanks stew for tea. Cooking duties was allocated to the person rostered off duty and this day, it was Peter's turn.

As Peter was serving the stew onto the plates, Paul yelled out, "What's this shit?"

Peter answered, "Lamb Shanks Stew."

Paul then yelled out, "Well I'm not eating this fucking dog shit. What do you think we are, fucking dogs?"

Paul then stormed out of the kitchen. As he walked out the rest of the crew went into a chorus of dog barking sounds. "Woof, Woof."

I set a simple rule at the dinner table: no criticism and comments if anyone didn't like the meals.

The next morning at around 3.00am I was awoken by the phone ringing. The OIC was the only person at Giles that had a phone in his donga (room), just in case of an emergency. I had been in a deep sleep and wondered who was ringing me at this time of the morning. It was Paul calling from the Met office. "Get your arse over here. I've been assaulted."

I was still half asleep. "What?" I replied. I couldn't believe what I has hearing.

Paul kept on rambling on the phone. "I've been assaulted by Peter. He's hit me in the face and head,"

Quickly I got dressed and headed to the Met Office and halfway I came across Peter drunk, stumbling and looking worse for wear.

Peter pointed to me and yelled out, "Dave, you can't prove a fucking thing. He fucking fell over."

I replied to Peter, "Get to bed and sleep it off."

On entering the Met office, Paul angrily pointed to his head and face. "This is what Peter did to me. He's king hit me in the face. He's drunk and came in and hit me. I want to lay charges." Looking at him, I could see his face was a real mess with his right eye heavily bruised and closed. Paul kept going on, "He just came in and hit me in the face without any reason. I hit my head on the floor. What are you fucking going to do about it?"

I came back to him. "Nothing. Serve you fucking right. Can you prove it?"

Paul loudly answered, "Of course I can. This is enough fucking proof."

I just couldn't be bothered with his problems and answered, "Where's your bloody witnesses? It's only your word against his. As far as I'm concerned you may have fallen over and hit your head and face in the dark somewhere."

Paul angrily replied, "You are fucking against me."

After I walked out of the Met office the incident was never mentioned again. I guess Paul knew that he had no witnesses or proof of Peter committing the assault. He had belittled me in front of people so my thinking was stuff him. Why should I help Paul with his poor attitude while he showed no respect for me and the other crew members? Good luck to Peter as, with my anger, I thought about hitting him many times myself.

Over a period of months at Giles, a lot of items disappeared including money from the Wongai hut canteen and from the Royal Flying Doctor charity box. Hans, our General Hand/

Mechanic, who looked after the money from the canteen and charity box had a strong suspicion that someone was knocking off the money! Unbeknown to me and other crew members he set a trap marking every $5 note that came into the canteen with a small 'x'. After a month he pulled the lever on the trap door by asking us if anybody had any small change including $5 dollar notes in exchange for $20 notes because he had run out of small change for the canteen. We all answered "no" except Paul, who answered he had a few $5 dollar notes that he brought in with him when he arrived at Giles and produced a roll of $5 notes. To Hans' shock, every $5 note Paul exchanged for $20 notes was marked "x".

Hans then fronted me about his trap.

> *I couldn't really do anything as I was not the law. I advised all to watch Paul and not let him work in the canteen by himself. As for the charity box, I arranged for Hans to solder a tin container together and that seemed to solve the problem as the only way to open it was with a can opener. For the other items such as tool kits and historic Giles memorabilia that disappeared and reappeared, Paul always knew where the missing items would turn up and be found after I threatened to call the Desert Patrol-Police to search each crew member's room. I always felt that Paul was the thief, but in the end, I couldn't prove a thing. What got me was it seemed to be a game for him to tell us where the missing items were.*

At times I felt like getting out of Giles on the first plane with the ongoing challenges and problems, but in the end the positives outweighed the negatives.

As we worked at Giles, we had permission to visit different areas of remote aborigine land, like Glen Cummings gorge, an oasis within it with freshwater rock pool, white ghost gum trees and spinifex grass.

A beautiful rugged gorge. To me it was like entering into another world, so quiet and peaceful.

Another special highlight for me was when I travelled on a dirt road to look at one of Len Beadell's bush signposts on a ghost gum tree near Schwerin Mura Crescent. Len Beadell was one of Australia's last great explorers in the 1950s and 60s. Len undertook solo surveys, graded and built roads through the outback and erected these aluminium-plated signposts throughout the expanses of the Western deserts.

Other great spots I visited were Surveyors General Corner where the Western Australia, South Australia and Northern Territory borders meet; the Rawlinson Range where we followed a track to the top by Land Rover and had spectacular views of Giles weather station on the open spinifex country with the distant white gum trees and desert oak on the open plains; the Red Sandy Desert via the Rawlinson Range and across the dry lakebed of Lake Christopher. The desert area we trekked through was mainly Spinifex, scrub and red sand dunes country.

Reality soon hit us about how dangerous this remote outback country was when our Land Rover got bogged in the thick red sand. We were never in danger as we always prepared for the odd mishap of breakdowns or being bogged. We had a CB (Citizens Band) radio in the vehicle, also shovels, mats, tools, and a winch up front of the Land Rover plus food tins and water-filled containers. First, we tried to use shovels and mats to get out but with no luck. We got out of the sand dune by using the winch attached to a nearby desert oak tree. On this trip we came across a lot of camels roaming the Red Sandy Desert.

My last trip was to Lasseter's cave about 42 kms from Docker River. Here Lewis Harold Bell Lasseter sheltered in the cave for approximately 25 days during January 1931. He had set out earlier with a herd of camels, to find a golden reef he claimed to have discovered 33 years earlier, but he became stranded in the cave without food after his camels bolted. Weak from starvation he died at Irving Creek 55 kms away from the cave as he tried to walk the 140 kms distance to Mt Olga assisted by a friendly aborigine family.

All up I felt privileged and lucky to be visiting these remote areas on aborigine land.

We had a lot of visitors and tourists over the six months at Giles including a Senator and his wife from Canberra, also State politicians and their aides who all stayed with us for a few nights. We also had a BBC television crew doing a documentary on the Australian outback and a journalist from the *Kalgoorlie Miner* newspaper who interviewed me about life at Giles.

The story was published in the Kalgoorlie Miner Weekender Saturday September 26th, 1998.

On one day in July we had 53 tourists through the Met Office. This was the peak of the busy tourist season. Most of the tourists travelled by 4WD, while others came through on tourist buses, cars, a few on motor bikes and even a couple on push bikes. We met all sorts and some real interesting characters. Most of the tourists were very friendly. They were interested in our work and lifestyle, in how we lived and coped in the isolated and remote area away from our families. We'd show them through the weather station and most times their visits would coincide with the release of the weather balloon. Beside the weather station there were other attractions for the tourists to see at Giles. Len Beadell's grader was in a cage built from strong wire mesh and covered with a corrugated iron roof. The grader was used to build the Gunbarrel Highway and other roads in the area. Len Beadell was also known as an artist and author. He had a couple of murals on the walls in our mess. We wouldn't advertise it to the tourists as it was in a private area for staff only, but some tourists knew about the murals and would ask us if they could view them. On most occasions we would oblige. The other big tourist attraction at Giles was the fenced exhibit of the remains of the Blue Streak Rocket which was launched from Woomera in June 1964 and discovered 50km southeast of Giles in 1980.

Meeting the tourists and visitors helped me to take my mind of the pressure of work and running the Weather Station.

For entertainment at Giles we all had our own interests and hobbies. I didn't have much time to relax as it was mainly work for me, but I did enjoy watching Aussie Rules Football matches on satellite TV and the latest video movies we ordered from a video store in Alice Springs that arrived weekly on the Ngaanyatjarra Air Flight.

On every Saturday night we had a barbecue night by the swimming pool. We usually invited the teachers, the nurses and the administrators from Warrakurna. At times we would attend their barbecues in at Warrakurna. At these barbecues, alcohol was not consumed or permitted outside on aborigine land, although we could drink alcohol inside our rooms or mess area.

The swimming pool, the barbecue area and the tennis court were known as the Country Club. "Country Club" was probably not an accurate name, as there was no alcohol allowed but I often enjoyed a swim in the pool when hot and it reminded me of an oasis in the middle of the desert.

My most depressing and unhappiest memory at Giles was on Saturday the 5th September.

It was the day when the Wongai hut was transported back to Warakurna and we had our last barbecue before heading home. It was the night of the big brawl between Hans, Peter and Paul. It all started when Hans and Peter accused Paul of knocking off money from the Wongai hut and his poor attitude. Fists went flying in all directions as Keith and I tried to break up the ugly brawl. Somehow, we managed to separate the three combatants and I thought all was calming down when Hans appeared with an iron bar in his hand that was used for smashing up glass. For the next frantic hostile second, I was in shock as the iron bar hurtled straight towards me and by a miracle missed by a few centimetres. In the hostile confusion Hans had mistakenly confused me with Paul who in the meantime had fled back to his room. Realising his horrible mistake, Hans couldn't have been more apologetic to me as he knew he could have killed me or inflicted a serious injury in his mad moment of rage.

For our last barbecue, the atmosphere was mournful and depressing. Only four of us turned up. Paul decided to take refuge in his room for the night, while Hans and Peter ended up drunk.

On the 7th September the new crew arrived by plane. They were lucky as they had a four-day changeover period compared to the one night I and my crew had. My last duty was to complete the stocktake of the station before handing over the responsibilities to the new OIC. On the 11th September, excited, I flew out of Giles for home.

Looking back now, it was a hard six months period, but I learnt a lot especially about myself and living in isolation with other people. I had no regrets, but I did miss my family. I didn't miss the busy world of suburban lifestyle, like shopping centres, road traffic, and workwise, answering endless incoming telephone calls, etc. I knew it was only a matter of time before I would apply for another remote posting because of my condition.

CHAPTER 22

BACK HOME AND FINALLY DIAGNOSED WITH PTSD

On my return home I took my family for a well earnt holiday for a week at Daydream Island in the Whitsunday group off the coast of Mackay.

After the holiday I returned to work at Rockhampton Met Office but soon I became unsettled again with anxiety and nightmares. My wife Deb was pressuring me to see a doctor, but it wasn't until I started going to a drop-in centre for veterans in Rockhampton that I realised it was past time to do something. The other vets could see my shakes and told me I had Post Traumatic Stress Disorder – Vietnam's calling card. After talking to them, I then went to see my local doctor and he referred me to a Psychiatrist Dr John Flanagan in Rockhampton. I was diagnosed with severe **PTSD – Post Traumatic Stress Disorder**. The doctor informed me that I had grounds to leave the workforce, particularly as my symptoms were so extreme.

> ***I was stubborn and blinded by my focus on escaping to isolation, so I ignored his recommendation. Taking his advice would be the easy way out.***

In early 1999 I applied for a position on Willis Island. It's located beyond the Great Barrier Reef in the Coral Sea, some 420 kms east of Cairns. Willis Island, like Giles, is a six months remote posting. I was successful for the OIC position and was to take up the position at the end of May. Unfortunately, I never did as my boy, David, broke his upper right arm in a freak accident at school by jumping from a balcony to the ground and landing awkwardly on his right shoulder. After David's accident I was in a quandary about leaving my family for six months. In the end I couldn't leave as it would have been selfish on my behalf and a lack of concern for my family, especially for David.

In March 2000 I decided to apply for a posting to Antarctica. In April I flew down to Melbourne for an interview with the Bureau of Meteorology selection committee for their Antarctica positions. It was a two-hour grilling from a three-person panel. I was successful but I first would have to pass a medical – physical and psychological examinations. In late April I fronted an Antarctic Division approved Psychiatrist at the Enoggera Army Base in Brisbane to answer questions and screened to ensure my mental health was suitable for remote isolation.

While he studied my every move searching for weaknesses, the Psychiatrist wasn't interested in my boyhood fantasies or thirst for adventure and challenges, he wanted to know about

Vietnam. "Tell me about Vietnam?" That was the question I'd been anxious about. The Vietnam veteran label had followed me around for years, as society learnt more about the scars on so many veterans. "Yeah, fine. A few nightmares, but nothing much. I don't drink much, nor smoke or do drugs. As far as I'm concerned, I'm fine. I've proven I can live in remote areas and isolation. In fact, I'm suited for it." That was all I was willing to say.

Somewhere in the back of my mind I knew that my anxiety attacks and nightmares weren't normal, but I figured that was my lot and I just wanted to get on with life. I'd gone to Giles to see how I'd cope with my nightmares and remoteness. I was confident that while PTSD was an issue for me, it wouldn't be an issue for anyone else and I wanted a challenge.

I must have convinced the Psychiatrist as a few days later I got the call that I was successful in all my medical checks and psych tests. I was expected in Hobart for training at the end of August to join the 2000-2001 expedition to Casey. In the meantime, I continued my shifts at Rockhampton.

I found it hard to focus on my duties and time seemed to drag on. Time wasn't dragging for my family. Before I'd applied, we had sat down together to discuss what it would mean to us if I pursued my dream. It would mean more than a year away at a time when Michelle and David would want me around for advice and support and leaving Deb to cope with everything by herself. I knew she was battling a sense of being left behind, an unfortunate reality for the families of expeditioners. However, it would also bring financial

benefits, especially with private school fees and university fees looming. Most importantly, it would mean an end to working at Rockhampton with its long commute and shift work.

In May one morning I was laying turf in the backyard when I felt pain in my groin area. After a few weeks the pain became severe and I felt unwell. I fronted my doctor and the news wasn't good. It was a hernia and would require an operation to fix it. The straight-forward operation went ahead in mid-June. My surgeon guaranteed I wouldn't be out of commission for too long, but my situation turned bad when they discovered in surgery that the hernia had strangulated a portion of my bowel.

I was a lucky boy. If I had left the operation any longer, it could have burst with fatal results.

Two weeks after the operation I went back to see my Surgeon for a follow-up examination. I was still bleeding from my bowel, so I knew the news wasn't going to be good. He sent me urgently to the Mater Private Hospital in Brisbane for a colonoscopy. It revealed 13 polyps in my bowel, the largest the size of a golf ball. The doctor removed the polyps during the colonoscopy procedure and sent the large one to a laboratory to determine if it was cancerous.

I went back to Yeppoon to wait for the results. I was finding it hard to remain optimistic. August was drawing near and the beginning of intensive ANARE – Australian National Antarctic Research Expeditions training. After an anxious week I received the good news it wasn't cancer.

I concentrated on getting fit and getting organised for August. In the meantime, my twin brother went in to have a colonoscopy, but they only found a couple of small polyps. The doctor believed my polyps could have been due to my Vietnam service since my twin brother hardly had any.

Two weeks before I was to depart for Hobart, I received a phone call. The professional voice at the other end introduced himself as Dr Peter Gormly, head of ANARE's medical division. After some small talk, he asked about my health.

Hoping it was a stock-standard question for all expeditioners, I answered in my usual manner: "Yeah, good."

He paused. "I believe you've been having some medical problems."

I knew neither of my doctors would've said anything and figured it must've been someone at the Rockhampton Meteorology office. I assumed he wouldn't know too many details. "Where'd you hear that? No, doc, I'm fine."

The doctor's tone changed, and he asked me again, this time telling me there was a Commonwealth Act which meant if I didn't tell the truth when questioned, there could be severe penalties. I thought I better tell him the truth. "I did have a hernia op in May, and they found a golf ball-sized polyp but I'm ok now."

Dr Gormly reply was shattering. "In that case, you're not going to Casey."

The last two months of worrying had finally come to this, and I wasn't going to back down. I argued with him, saying that both my doctors said I'd be medically fit by August. Dr Gormly replied I would need medical certificates from them both before I went to Hobart and he left it at that. I sent the two medical certificates from my doctors to ANARE Hobart, stating I was medically fit.

CHAPTER 23

THE BEGINNING OF THE CURSE OF CASEY

Saying goodbye to Deb, Michelle and David was hard.

> ***On the trip down to Hobart I was hollow, questioning the fairness of what I was doing, especially as my kids were at an age when they should have their dad nearby.***

At the Antarctica Division's building in Kingston Hobart, I met the other 20 expeditioners who were also to head down to Casey. One introduced himself as the station's doctor and said he wanted to talk to me. What he wanted to do was medically examine me. Afterwards he said: "I'm not happy to take you, Dave. I just don't want the risk." I froze. Surely, I wasn't going to be turned away now, after I arrived. I argued I was fit and had two medical certificates from my two doctors to confirm this. The final decision was made by Dr Gormly that I would not go to Casey and I was immediately dismissed from the ANARE training program.

> *I was devastated and angry. I couldn't understand why after I had organised the medical certificates, left work, said goodbye to my family, travelled to Hobart and then they finally decided to send me home. Couldn't they have made that decision before I left?*

The disappointment of the aborted Casey expedition rested heavily as I forced myself to go back to work. I couldn't cope with the stress and pressure and found it difficult taking phone calls from the public.

My family suggested I should take a break from work and go on leave. I did that as I had accumulated enough leave over time. We decided to go to America and visit Ron, Sandy and their girls in Helena, Montana. We experienced our first white Christmas together and I thought this was what it would look like in Antarctica with snow and blizzard conditions.

After six weeks leave, I was back at work in Rockhampton and preparing a new application form to Antarctica when in March 2001, I received a phone call from the head of the ANARE Meteorology program asking if I was interested in going to Macca – Macquarie Island – for six months. Apparently pulling me out from Casey had caused a problem with station postings. The Met person who was due to head to Macquarie Island had filled my position at Casey while the Macquarie Island position was filled short term for the winter period only. Now they needed someone to fill the 2001 Officer-in-Charge summer season role.

I'd immediately said yes. I wasn't going to knock back a chance to get my foot through the door to get to one of the Antarctica stations. I was now fully recovered and couldn't believe my luck. Once again, I had to prepare my family for a seven-month separation. They supported my decision and sympathised with me over what had happened in Hobart.

At home on the 18th July I answered a phone call from a distressed David, asking me to pick him up from school. When I arrived at the school at around 5pm, he was emotionally upset. David told me he had been physically assaulted by his Religious teacher and pointed out visible bruises on his chest and neck area. David was doing community service for a four-day period and had to stay in the school dormitory overnight during this period. After completing the community service for the day at around 2.30pm, David and a group of boys arrived back at school early and proceeded to the dormitory. The rules were the dormitory was out of bounds to all students until after 3pm. While they were in the dormitory, a lady supervisor approached them in an impatient manner and wanted them to leave. David questioned her "Why" and this apparently upset the supervisor. After she contacted someone on the phone, she then ordered David to report to a teacher at the school library. David proceeded to the library and just before he reached the library near a garden area, he was confronted by his Religious education teacher.

Note: I have taken the following information from the Police Witness Statement reported by David on the 20th July 2001.

David's Religious teacher approached him and pointed to the garden area. "Get over there. Who do you think you are?" "How dare you abuse my wife." At the same time he grabbed the top of David's shirt and collar area as well as his tie. "You better be careful or else I will knock your head in." David felt pain around the throat area and nearly tripped backwards over rocks into the garden as the teacher forcefully pushed and held David tightly around the throat in a throttling motion. David, emotionally stressed, kept on saying "Let me go, you are hurting me." The teacher then took David to the administration office where David had to front the Deputy Principal. Once in the office the Religious teacher told the Deputy Principle what had happened, then David told his side of the incident and had to write out a statement but in the end they seemed not interested about the assault.

I was fuming and upset and fronted the Head Principal that evening with David. The Head Principal, a Brother of the Private Religious school, had a bad reputation. He was well known in Queensland for his outlandish behaviour in discipling students. My Vietnam mate, Col Hegarty in Townsville and our BOM Rockhampton Technician had warned me beforehand about his reputation for using outrageous methods. At the meeting I showed the Principal David's bruised chest and neck area and I asked him what steps he was going to take to discipline the teacher. He was not interested and stated it was David's fault for being rude to the teacher's wife. The conversation became heated when the Principal started pointing his finger at me and David. "You are a poor parent and the rudest parent I have ever met, and your son is not much better than you. I guarantee your son will fail in life and be in jail by the time he reaches twenty-one."

I remember those humiliating horrible toxic words to this day and my reply. "Do not judge me and my son, judge yourself. Your organisation has a repeated history of protecting sexual and physical offenders so judge them."

All this, blaming David and protecting the coward teacher triggered all my **anger** symptoms within me. I felt like smashing his face in but somehow I resisted the temptation. My final words, "You will all hear from my solicitor." We then walked out of the office. David went to see his doctor the next day where the doctor observed and noted his injuries and on the 20th he submitted a witness statement on the assault to the Yeppoon Police Station. On the 25th July David and I visited a solicitor in Rockhampton to act against the teacher.

We had a substantial case against the teacher until our witnesses, David's mates, started to pull out because the parents did not want to get involved due to the repercussions their sons faced if they gave evidence which might impact their education.

I was shattered by that outcome and ruminated for weeks about how I would get justice and revenge for David but in the end I believe the teacher would have spent many sleepless nights worrying about the impending assault charge. In summing up David's attitude, I believe he has an extraordinarily strong character as many teenagers at his age would have given school away and struggled with life but he showed them up with a top career and is now a Senior Civil Engineer with 12 years design and construction experience on civil, transportation and tunnel projects in Australia, Canada, United Kingdom, and New Zealand.

Success is the best form of revenge.

CHAPTER 24

MACQUARIE ISLAND

On 2nd September I left Rockhampton for Melbourne to do training at the Bureau's training school.

> ***Another emotional goodbye at the airport. It wasn't any easier the second time around.***

I needed training in the Ozone-sondes used at Macca – the only Sub-Antarctic site to launch them. This balloon-borne device profiles ozone concentration from the ground up to an altitude of about 35 kilometres and measures the ozone concentration of the sampled air. A standard meteorological radiosonde is incorporated in the balloon payload, and provides additional data on pressure, temperature and humidity every 10 seconds during the flight. An onboard global positioning systems (GPS) receiver provides location information.

After three days training in Melbourne I flew out to Hobart for more training and to be kitted out with gear.

On the morning of 12th September I flicked on the television and stared at the screen before realising I was watching Armageddon. Planes slammed into buildings, people jumped from incomprehensible heights, white ghosts calmly walked out of the city in shock. September 11 in America was chaos as terrorists attacked New York's Twin Towers.

> *I rang my family, who were also watching, and we tried to make sense of what was happening. We couldn't, although we sensed its impact. It was raw and unprocessed, and it stunned us. I spent hours watching "America Under Attack". I watched the Towers collapse repeatedly on the screen and I recalled visiting them in 1975. My disbelief and terrible sadness for the families whose worlds had been shattered left me with an overwhelming need to be with my family. It didn't escape me that I was about to put even more distance between us.*

Further training followed, including three days of forklift training and four days of field training at Bronte Park Highland Village, located midway between Hobart and Queenstown in the geographic centre of Tasmania. Expeditioners need a wide range of skills to work at the stations and it was mandatory to undergo the four-day pre-departure training. The first two days we spent out in the field and trained on navigation, compass skills, radios, and search and rescue.

> *Night-time had become my enemy. I had to share a tent with another expeditioner for two nights and I had to warn him of my nightmares. In the end I didn't have any nightmares – I couldn't sleep as my tent mate snored heavily during the night.*

CHAPTER 24

The final two days back at the Village we had classroom sessions on environmental management, coping with separation from family and friends, occupational health and safety, harassment and issues with community living. Our last training session was on the four-wheel-drive Honda quad bikes and finally, there was a formal dinner and drinks session with all the ANARE executives.

Last day back in Hobart I had to attend the Tasmania Fire training school at Cambridge. It was hard physical work, rolling and unrolling hoses and setting up equipment.

On the 28th September I boarded the bright orange icebreaker, *Aurora Australis* (AA), affectionately known as the "Orange Roughy". Named for the southern hemisphere's night phenomenon, she's Australia's Antarctic flagship, and was purposely built for the program by P&O Polar. The ship accommodates 116 passengers, and at 94 metres long and 3911 tonnes, can break ice up to 1.5 metres thick. Three helicopters can be housed in the hanger and operate from the deck at the rear of the ship.

After safety drills, at 6.30pm the ship's horn blasted, and we pulled away. Thin paper streamers connecting expeditioners with their loved ones on the wharf snapped one by one until finally we were on our own.

> ***My family wanted to fly down to Hobart to see me off. I refused as I couldn't handle the intensity of my feelings in saying goodbye. In the end I knew my decision was right as it was gut-wrenching watching others say goodbye.***

Cold, wet and windy, Macquarie Island ("Macca") rises from

the Southern Ocean about 1500 kilometres south south-east of Tasmania, halfway between Australia and Antarctica. After a long history of sealing, it became a nature reserve under the control of the Tasmanian government and is now a breeding refuge for southern elephant seals, fur seals and penguins. Approximately 34 kilometres long by 5.5 kilometres at its widest point, it became a World Heritage area in 1997.

The island is beautiful and rugged. It poked up through the mist at 11.30am after three day's journey from Hobart. I gathered on the deck with others to stare at the desolate cragginess which would be home for the next six months. I was desperate to get off the "Orange Roughy" as the Southern Ocean had served her reputation well. I had spent the better part of the journey with my head in a toilet bowl due to the rough seas.

The captain dashed my hopes, announcing the 20-25 knot winds and white-capped water meant we'd have to keep moving down the east side of the island, 34 kilometres to the southern Hurd Point area and wait for better conditions. I wasn't prepared for the wild beauty as we sailed past massive clusters of penguin colonies and seemingly comatose elephant seals dotted in the distance on pebbled beaches. Behind the beaches the land rose sharply to the plateau upland. After a few hours and in better weather conditions we returned to Buckles Bay about a kilometre offshore. Soon afterwards, I arrived on the Island by zodiac boat and was greeted by the Station leader Robb Clifton and outgoing BOM officer-in-charge.

Normally the changeover period lasts for four days however this one lasted for fifteen minutes. The outgoing officer-in-charge only had enough time to show me the office, the diary and hand me the keys before he rushed off to get onto the ship. I was taking over the Met Station like "Blind Freddy". I was fortunate I had an experienced BOM Technician in Cathie whom I first met at Giles when she came out to fix our equipment.

The first night at Macca I had a bad nightmare, screaming out with my body shaking uncontrollably and gasping for breath.

I had nightmares when I was in unfamiliar surroundings.

I was lucky having only one occupied room next to me while the other room was the main toilet and shower/laundry room.

The next few days I worked at the Met office to learn my new role with help from Cathie and Ailsa. The Met office ran two shifts: 8am-4pm and 4pm-12.30am. Each shift had specific duties, including releasing a weather balloon and three stages for an Ozone balloon release. Other duties were to change filters and pump air through cylinders at the Clean Air Laboratory building with the data sent to various universities and the CSIRO – Commonwealth Scientific and Industrial Research Organisation.

All the bases in Antarctica have a well-established roster service for domestic chores. Every day one person, "Baywatch", does morning cleaning and another, "Slushie", does kitchen duties like scrubbing pots, cleaning floors, peeling potatoes and wiping tables. On Saturday mornings everyone was allotted other duties like cleaning different areas of the station, garbage runs and restocking supplies.

For entertainment, Saturday night was the major social night of the week with possibly a themed night where you could dress up and let loose.

Everyone had to do field training as soon as they arrived at any ANARE station. I was looking forward to seeing the island outside of the station confines and the challenge of the training itself. Finally, after three weeks it was my turn along with three others as we headed off with Field Training Officer Christian Gallagher, nickname Psycho. On any trip from the station you always had to take a VHF radio and map, and everything packed into plastic bags because of the wet climate. From Gadget Gully we climbed up to the plateau. I'd thought I was fit, but it didn't take long for my body to convince me otherwise. As I crawled up the rocks, my back and legs were screaming out with pain from the weight of clothes, bivvy bag, survival food and water. Everyone was struggling both physically and mentally except Psycho. When we got to the top, the spectacular view down to the isthmus and across to the Nuggets momentarily silenced my aching body. Psycho cheerily told us we had a further five kilometres to go across the plateau before we could rest at the field hut at Bauer Bay. After a gut-wrenching walk, at times through featherbed vegetation, we arrived late afternoon at the corrugated iron shed with a small veranda surrounded by tussock grass.

By now my back was strained and I could hardly put one foot in front of the other.

We still had more training to do hopping into a bivvy bag. A bivvy bag is used to prevent hypothermia when someone is caught out in cold freezing blizzard conditions and unable to build emergency shelter. It is designed to conserve energy and body heat. The theory is to get into a wind-free area, either behind a rock or even the slightest depression in the ground and wait it out. Basically, you bury yourself in a bag with a small vent opened.

I wriggled into the bivvy bag and fell into a deep sleep for a few short minutes before a nightmare hit me. Screaming I thought I was back in Vietnam buried in the pit hole. I thrashed in the bag until I got my head out and realisation hit. Shaking and gasping I couldn't fully put my head back in. After about ten minutes Psycho told me to go to the hut.

Inside the hut we relaxed in the cosy heat and had a meal. Psycho gave my legs a rub down as my body calmed.

When expeditioners ventured to the huts on the Island, we used the ocean for our toilet like Mother Nature intended. Going to the toilet during the night I had to cautiously scope the area for seals.

After a restful night, the next day was like the first day. The navigation and medical training continued as we trudged four kilometres back across the Island to the east coast to Sandy Bay and walked along the beach to a hut at Brothers Point. The red apple-shaped hut, known as an igloo satellite cabin, was made of fibreglass and fully insulated with double glazed polycarbonate windows. The alien-looking shelter was nestled in a green valley close to the ocean with stunning views. Huddled in the tiny "red apple" we settled for the night and chatted, exchanging stories on family, our life stories and how we ended up at Macca.

I felt a sense of camaraderie like I did in the Army.

The next morning, our final day and by far the hardest, we headed back up the island towards base, into the famous Macca wind. Gusts up to 90 kilometres per hour toyed with us, pushing us back one step for each two we took forward. The nine-kilometre trek took us six hours to complete. The rain cut our visibility and made heavy work of slogging through the wet sand.

At the Nuggets we slid over the rocks and pebbles before a treacherous climb in from the sea, up a rock cliff and along a narrow walkway. I hugged the cliff side, fighting the wind's attempts to pick me up and throw me over. Psycho calmly warned us if that happened, we should try and land in the sea on our backs so the packs would cushion the fall. As we struggled towards the base, finally the station appeared in the distance teasing us until we got close enough, to be sure it was real.

> ***My aching body was rewarded with a hot shower and clean clothes. I can honestly say it was my hardest walk since my Army rookie training days at Kapooka when on a twenty kilometres forced march, I ended up with massive blisters on both of my feet.***

People's characters had started to become clearer, and cracks had begun to show among some of the expeditioners' relationships. Isolation, both geographic and from friends and family, brought frustrations which began to spark clashes. As a summer expeditioner it took a while to notice that there was an undercurrent among some of the winter expeditioners. As the officer-in-charge of the Met program, I'd tried to resolve problems between Ailsa and Cathie. They had come in as friends, but different values and lifestyle choices had caused tension which often broke out under the guise of work issues. Complaints like ozone-sondes not being properly prepared and corners cut on shift duties would often cause arguments between them. I tried to mediate and resolve the girl's differences but couldn't. Despite everyone's best efforts, Ailsa decided to leave the Island and return to Australia in early December on the tourist ship *Akademik shokalski*.

> ***I knew her departure would have a big impact on the Met program. Cathie and I would have to split Ailsa's work between us for the remainder of the season.***

I also had to take over the store position, supplying any clothing needs required by the expeditioners and restocking huts by zodiac boat. To me it was a positive, getting out on the ocean and restocking huts as it was a chance to see the Island. Whenever we needed to head out on the ocean, the rule was a minimum of two zodiacs with at least two people in each one. We had to carry radios, bivvy bags and other essential gear in case the weather turned bad and forced us to stay in one of the huts overnight along the coast.

Often, we were joined in the zodiacs by the elephant seal program team scanning the ocean for seals with time-depth data recorder units attached to the backs of female and juvenile seals to record their foraging habits. At times along the way we would stop the zodiac so the seal team could set up their antenna and sweep back and forth in search of any signal transmissions.

I also got involved in the fur seal program where I'd help the team by weighing, measuring, and taking biopsies from recently born pups. It was dangerous work as we had to watch out for the dominant aggressive bulls. After each well-performed routine, we would mark the pup with a number. The breeding numbers were being monitored.

With work and the priceless opportunity to explore the Island, time went quickly. Before I knew it, we were celebrating Christmas and New year. The festivities for Christmas lifted everyone's mood as we exchanged gifts followed by the traditional Christmas dinner with all sorts of food including oysters, smoked salmon, crayfish, king prawns, turkey, ham, pork, roast vegies, salads, bread rolls and for desert, plum pudding, ice cream and Christmas cake.

An exquisite Christmas feast was accompanied by eggnog and an unlimited selection of reds, whites, beer, cider, ports, champagne and spirits.

> ***It was a Christmas feast I will never forget but the most significant and meaningful part of Christmas for me is being with my family. This was my first Christmas away from Deb, Michelle and David. I rang my family and listened to them describing their day. I missed them. Christmas is all about family, and we weren't together to share the joy.***

For New Year we gathered on the Station Leader's hut patio for a spit roast lamb and barbecue. After eating we gathered around a bonfire prepared nearby earlier in the day, where we chatted and toasted in the new year, 2002, in.

> ***It was easily the most unusual place that I'd finished a year out.***

I sought out Robb, Station Leader, for some advice. I'd been encountering hostility from a fellow expeditioner, who was a friend when I arrived at Macca. About my age, we'd spent quite a bit of time chatting at the bar, laughing and enjoying a growing friendship. I knew he'd had some personal problems before coming down to Macca, a bitter divorce scarring his view on relationships. Then one night, while sitting at the bar chatting with him, one of the female expeditioners asked me to join the others in a dance. It seemed to upset him. The next time I sat down next to him in the mess, he grunted, picked up his plate and left. He didn't speak to me again. The tension of living in close quarters with this hostility was getting to me. I talked it over with Robb and asked him if he could approach this person to find out his problem with me.

> *I usually do not involve others in my problems, but I trusted Robb. An ex-SAS officer, he was a good leader, very calm and collected. Above all he knew how to handle all sorts of people and I never saw him lose it once. Robb said he'd have a word with him and get us together to resolve the problem.*

The 18th January was a day I will never forget. It started well enough, with three teams heading out to resupply the huts at Brothers Point, Green Gorge, on the east coast and Hurd Point at the bottom of the Island.

The teams consisted of two in each of the zodiacs. The first zodiac boat launched into the water carried me and Cal. Psycho and Paul were in the second and Gerbil and Robbo in the third. The trip was relatively calm, and penguins kept us company along the way down the coast as we supplied huts at Brothers Point and

Green Gorge. At Green Gorge we picked up some rocks from a geologist. As we travelled further south the weather started to turn with winds picking up to around 25 knots and the seas rising to three metres. The leader of the boating party decided to keep going, but by then it was hard to see the other boats over the waves. With the wind howling, I started to feel uneasy. I carefully wrapped my video camera into a waterproof bag and tucked it away into a safety pocket of the zodiac. At Hurd Point our zodiac was the first to attempt to catch a wave into shore. A huge wave caught us and flipped us into the dangerous rough waters.

I am not a strong swimmer, so I thought this is it and I accepted my fate.

I could hear others yelling, "Where's Dave?" My beanie had slipped over my face and I was trapped in the swirling water under the zodiac. I struggled and somehow surfaced from under the zodiac, shoving my beanie away. I could see Cal still attached to the zodiac. Gasping for breath, my lungs burning, I felt time slowed as a second large wave picked us up and slammed us into rocks. Choking on water, I grabbed onto what I could, but a strong rip pulled us back out into deep, swirling water. My chest was burning, and I kept gasping for breath, desperate for sweet air among the claustrophobic water.

A powerful third wave approached, picked us up and luckily spat us out on the beach. Cal and I stumbled across the hard sand and pebbles, dragging what was left of the zodiac onto the shore. We collapsed with our dry suits pulling tight and deep cuts stinging from the salty water. Cal was bleeding from the head.

Shock and exhaustion silenced us. Psycho and Paul managed to ride in safely on a big wave, but Gerbil and Robbo's boat flipped. Their wave was kinder, bringing them onto the beach straight past the rocks. We lost all the supplies as well as our only radio plus the rocks in the two zodiacs that flipped.

Our boat was ruined. We sat in shock and stared at the wreck in disbelief. The waves and the chatter of thousands of surrounding penguins were the only sounds. Finally, someone spoke. "Well, what do we do now?" It was decided three of us would go in each of the two remaining zodiacs, plus what we could salvage from the beach. We decided to take the motor from the wrecked zodiac and leave the shell behind. Cal was by far the strongest swimmer and we decided he would help launch the zodiacs before swimming out through the breaking waves to his boat. Studying the waves, we counted a 15-second gap between them. Psycho and Paul went first, with all of us pushing their zodiac into the swirling water. They timed the waves, gunned the motor, and pushed over a series of big waves to be successful on their first attempt. It was our turn with Cal, Gerbil, Robbo, and I pushing the second zodiac out. Cal pushed as we jumped in, and Gerbil tried frantically to start the motor. Just as he got the motor started, the tiny window of opportunity closed. We got picked up and flipped over into the angry water and luckily the wave pushed us straight past the rocks onto the beach. "This is a bloody joke," I said to Gerbil, trembling with cold and panic.

I was thinking I would rather walk the 34 kilometres back to base than try again. I stared at the waves frustrated and feeling terrified. I was living a nightmare in the middle of the day but I knew I had no option but to join the others.

We started pushing the boat back out again, fighting to keep it straight against the movement of the water. I was up to my shoulders in the icy water and struggled to lift my body through the heavy water into the zodiac. Robbo heaved me in as Gerbil struggled with the motor again but this time it roared to life and we successfully managed to get over the dangerous breaking big waves. We pulled alongside the other zodiac and waited for Cal. The waves were picking us up and dropping us down so far that Hurd Point would disappear entirely for a few seconds until we rose again. Cal successfully swam back to the other zodiac despite finding it difficult at times swimming through thick patches of kelp.

The return trip to the station was slow as we had to pick up a science person who flagged us down from one of the huts. After re-arranging the zodiacs once again, we crept back to the base overloaded with four people in one zodiac and three plus remaining supplies in the other.

We finally returned to the station late that afternoon, four hours behind schedule and feeling sore, bruised, and sunburnt. Robb, the Station leader, met us and was relieved to see we had all survived.

I was heading back to have a hot shower desperate to ease my aches and pains when I was fronted by the expeditioner I was having trouble with. "I want to see you. I'm fuckin' sick of you. So when can I fuckin' see you?" he snarled, poking a finger at my face. Apparently, Robb fronted him earlier at my request.

The adrenalin and fear of the past few hours had left me with an emotional hollowness.

"You'll have to wait. I am going to have a shower, then we can talk. I'll meet you in the Met office shortly," I replied, walking past him. After my shower I went to the Met office and waited. It took a while to realise he was not going to show.

> *Robb was disappointed with the outcome. I was not interested in confronting him about our issues again especially as we only had six weeks to go before we departed Macca.*

The next day we had a big debrief with Robb about the accident. Several recommendations and instructions were instigated: a requirement to turn back if the weather became uncertain; having an observer at Hurd Point advising by radio on the weather conditions; and no beaching by boat allowed at Hurd Point unless there was someone at the hut.

> *There have been several periods in my life where I faced fear. The boating accident had increased my symptoms of PTSD especially with anxiety.*
>
> *There are factors that can generate high levels of anxiety over time after traumatic events. In my case: –*
>
> *Emotions – anxious, stressed, fearful, worried, feelings of panic, on edge, apprehensive, restless, overwhelmed, unreal and sense of impending doom.*
>
> *Thinking – negative, poor concentration at times, and catastrophising how I will cope.*
>
> *Behaviour – Withdrawal, isolation. Avoidance, escape. Confrontation, aggression. Agitation, unable to relax.*
>
> *Physical – trembling/shaking, sweating, sleep difficulties,*

fatigue/exhaustion, rapid heartbeat, shortness of breath, nausea, dizziness, restlessness, and headaches.

A few days later I had the chance to head back out on the water for another run down the coast. As I climbed in the Zodiac, I checked myself for any nerves and was surprised to find I was okay. We headed down to Green Gorge and unloaded supplies then back up to Brothers Point to continue our supply.

Earthquakes at Macquarie are a regular occurrence. I experienced two while there. The first was in the pitch black of the night while asleep. I thought I was having a nightmare but realised the terror was a tremor as I jumped out of bed. The second occurred while at work in the late afternoon. I hung onto the desk while the office shook and the noise was an incredible roar. Like the first, the quake measured around 5.3 on the Richter scale, the epicentre 40 kilometres away and 10 kilometres deep.

It was the beginning of the end. The station was preparing for the end of the summer season and the arrival of the 'AA'- *Aurora Australis* Voyage 8 (V8), in a couple weeks bringing in the new winter crew and supplies to the station.

The 'AA' was behind schedule due to mechanical problems. The delayed changeover meant a lot of smokers were caught out with no cigarettes. For a while they were scrounging from each other until all ran out. One bright young spark expeditioner collected tobacco from old butts from the ashtrays and bins and turned them into normal cigarettes. Until the AA arrived, every late afternoon and evening on the mess veranda, at least half a dozen desperate smokers worked in a production line to produce a new brand of cigarette to satisfy their cravings.

After the night of our big end-of-summer-expedition party, we woke the next morning, to find, shimmering in the morning light, the *Aurora Australis* anchored in Buckles Bay. The next six days from sun-up to sunset were organized chaos with incoming supplies transported from the 'AA' by a six-wheel-drive amphibious vehicle known as a 'Duck' and by helicopters. I had to brief the new Met crew regarding duties required on each shift and my tips after six month's experience.

On the final Saturday night, we gathered in the mess for both a farewell and welcome party.

It was a heavy night, and very crowded with sixty odd people crammed in.

> ***I could not take it, felt invaded so went back to the solitude of my room. My shakes were visible as my body tried to cope with the anxiety of the crowd. Even one of the new expeditioners questioned me about my shakes. There was a rumour going around that I was a drunk as the new arrivals had seen my shakes and they assumed I was an alcoholic going through withdrawals or waiting for my next drink.***

Finally, on the 19th March we were ready. The day was miserable, with heavy snow showers and hail. I rang Deb and the kids and told them I was about to depart, and I would call them when I arrived in Hobart in three days' time.

Having the helicopters flying back and forth over my head for days had been bad enough, but now I was going to have to climb into one. Psycho knew my background and what I was going through. He got me in and nodded to the pilot to start his lift off procedure.

Getting into the helicopter was the hardest. Once the helicopter lifted and gained height, I was ok.

Looking down at the craggy beauty of the Island's coastline and the buildings dotted along the edge of the isthmus was so different from what I always remembered seeing from a chopper – ***flashbacks of Vietnam.***

The trip over to the AA was short, probably two minutes at the most, and the helicopter settled gracefully onto the helipad deck. At 7.30pm, the ship's horn sounded three short toots. We gathered at the stern and lit flares, and at the distant base they did likewise. I heard someone say, "That's the finish then". And it was. I watched the outline of the station become smaller and felt emotional.

The island was special with its different animals, the rugged beauty of the land, and the ever-changing climate.

The next few days were a blur for me as seasickness took hold. On the morning of the 22nd after five months and twenty days away I arrived back at Macquarie Dock in Hobart. There were feelings of excitement as Macca expeditioners were reunited with their families.

I asked Deb and the kids not to meet me in Hobart, as emotional public reunions are not my style. I wanted space and privacy in greeting them.

I had a few chores to take care of before I could go home. In the afternoon I had the official debriefing with the Regional bosses in which I had to go over all the issues I had experienced at Macca. They congratulated me on doing an outstanding job for the six months. At the same time, my other priority was to submit my application form for the 2003 Antarctica expedition at one of the Australian bases on the ice.

The next morning, I left Hobart. The day was a blur of flights to Melbourne, then to Brisbane and finally to Rockhampton where my family greeted me. It was overwhelming to finally hold Deb, Michelle, and David and to find them all happy and healthy.

For now, I was home in Yeppoon. That was all that mattered to me.

I tried to get back to the real world again, but I struggled with the loss of the safe confines of the station and the camaraderie of the other expeditioners.

Once again, I found myself a changed man in a world that had not changed. The last time I felt like this was when I left the pungent jungle and climbed on the "Freedom Bird" back to Australia.

After five weeks' leave, I returned to work at Rockhampton Met Office but found it hard to adjust to the daily routine of shift work. The weeks passed expecting a phone call from the Antarctica Division on my application. Instead I got a phone call from Cathie, the Met Technician I had worked with at Macca asking me what happened to my application for Antarctica as the Met staff for 2003 ANARE – Australian National Antarctic Research Expeditions had all been chosen. I froze, I could not believe it. I immediately rang the boss of the Met Antarctica program and he was shocked to hear that I had applied for the 2003 program when I submitted when I arrived back from Macca. Further investigation eventually found my application form at the bottom of a drawer under a pile of paperwork.

It was a major stuff up. I rang the Union representative who told me the Bureau would have to recall all applications and resit interviews again for a fair process with the rules treating all applicants equally without favouritism or discrimination.

This was confirmed by the Regional Director in Hobart, that they would have to go through the process again. A few days later I answered a call from him offering me work at Davis Base on OIC wages but working under the original selected OIC.

He stated it would cost a huge amount of money and time for the Bureau to interview all applicants again and this was by far the best way to solve the whole problem. He told me it was more likely I would have been selected to Casey Base as the OIC.

Curse of Casey? I wondered if I was cursed to get down to Casey as this was the second time I had tried.

My main priority was to get down on the Ice, so I had no hesitation in accepting the deal and in fact it was a bonus for me as I had less responsibility but still OIC wages. I knew the selected OIC in Geoff Fulton (Beacon) who was a mate of mine and I worked previously with him. Also, a plus, a few of the Macca crew I had served with were selected for Davis: Cathie the Met Technician, Cal the Deputy leader/plumber and our cook Gerbil.

June was busy with a medical exam in Rockhampton then a trip to Brisbane for the psych test at Enoggera Army Barracks.

Soon afterwards I got a call from the Met Antarctica program boss asking me about the guy who I had fallen out with while down at Macca. He then dropped a bomb shell. “Guess what? He’s going down to Davis with you.” I was shocked. I could not believe what he was saying. My reply, “If that’s the case, the Antarctica Division will have to get us together and help us talk our problems through, otherwise there is no way we can work together for twelve months.”

Cal the Deputy leader down at Macca with me heard about the guy being posted to Davis as well. Like me he did not get on with him, so he contacted the ANARE Division and voiced his opinion. After two weeks I was relieved when told ANARE had decided to post the guy to Casey instead.

CHAPTER 25

DAVIS BASE ANTARCTICA

At the beginning of August, I was on my way, again leaving my family. Michelle was now at University and David in Year 12. Deb was dreading becoming a "Met widow" again. She worked part-time at the local school doing intervention work, helping students who were struggling with learning.

> ***With training and time at Davis I would be away for a total of 15 months, much longer than my seven-month stints at Giles and Macca. I consoled myself that this was not my final goodbye, that I would try to get back for a few days after completing the training and before the ship departed.***

Training covered a range of outcomes. Firstly a few days in Melbourne with Met training and then onto Hobart for the Basic ANARE training. I was required to do fire-fighting training, a gymnasium course, and as I had volunteered to be one of the hairdressers, I attended a hairdresser's course at the Hobart TAFE (Technical and Further Education). I was also on the hydroponics team and sat through an introduction course on how to grow fresh vegetables.

The Davis station leader, Jeremy Smith, had chosen me to train up as a scrub nurse to assist the station doctor in any emergency critical situation while we were down at Davis. Four expeditioners were chosen to train, two as scrub nurses and two as anaesthesiologists at the Royal Hobart Hospital for two weeks. I learnt to perform a range of duties from cleaning and caring for the instruments, performing the roles of scout or scrub nurse in surgery, to meeting the physical and emotional needs of the patient, maintaining airways and observing and monitoring a patient's vital signs in a recovery room.

In the days leading up to the start of the course, I started suffering anxiety about how I would handle it as I had seen enough blood and trauma while in Vietnam. It was daunting, but I knew this was a tried and tested method and that I had to trust the system.

The first day at the hospital was tense. Jim Milne, the other expeditioner selected, and I learnt how to scrub, glove and gown, maintaining a sterile and controlled atmosphere. Doing that was critical and the steps to each skill were drummed into us.

I forced myself to take deep breaths and focus on what the Perioperative Clinical Educator was saying.

The first week of training included instrument handling, positioning of patients, and surgical count – a legal requirement of any operation, no matter how minor. We practised until everything became routine. The week finished with a mock exercise: going in, washing, gloving up, gowning, and ensuring sterility.

On the weekend my brain became numb as I mentally reviewed all the steps and details. We were going to step into a live theatre on the Monday, and my anxiety was building, triggering nightmares and flashbacks again.

On Monday morning I told the Perioperative Clinical Educator Di Beamish my background, needing her to understand where I was coming from before I set foot in an operating theatre. Telling Di relieved some of the anxiety.

"Don't worry. There have been people in the past who have fainted, and I promise I will be with you," she said.

After they scrubbed and gowned me, I entered the operating theatre, I was numb.

When the surgeon cut the patient's stomach open, I was amazed I felt no emotions, no feelings whatsoever and accepted the blood on the gloves.

For the rest of the week I assisted in all sorts of operations under strict supervision. It was a very regimented atmosphere, from the instrument handling to the count of instruments. My most memorable experience in the theatre was helping the doctors and nurses deliver a baby girl by caesarean.

Each time, the scrubbing, gowning and preparation became easier, and I was slowly becoming more confident.

CHAPTER 25

The Royal Hobart Hospital, a respected teaching hospital, was the only hospital in Australia to train Antarctic expeditioners and they were proud of it. That pride was obvious to us with all the doctors, nurses, and staff positive, helpful, and supportive of us.

The final training was another stint at Bronte Park where survival was drilled, and redrilled into us. Field training is mandatory for each expeditioner heading to an Antarctica station.

Social nights and time off broke the intensity of training. All the Davis expeditioners attended meetings mainly at pubs so we could get to know each other and bond together having meals and drinks.

I watched hell unfold on 12th October when the Bali bombings occurred. This time it was people stumbling out of the popular Sari Club and Paddy's in Bali. All up, 202 people died in the terrorist bombings, including 88 Australians with a further 209 injured. It was the second time I had turned on the television and witnessed terrorism before I headed south on an expedition. The last time was before I went to Macca when terrorists attacked New York's Twin Towers on September 11, 2001.

After Bronte Park we were given a week off before the ship departed. I took the opportunity to go home to visit my family. It was good to see them but disturbing in some ways as I could not settle down and my emotions were high. Time passed so quickly and before I knew it, I was on a flight back to Hobart.

> ***My thinking in going home was it would be a twelve-month absence from my family instead of fifteen if I did not go home.***

People questioned my behaviour in continuing to leave my family. Was it because I was selfish and it was all about myself or was it that I did not care about my family? It was neither. It was about my PTSD – I sought isolation. I had become obsessed with it; in fact, it was like a drug to me. Behaviour: Withdrawal, isolation. Avoidance, escape.

At 6pm on November 22nd the *Aurora Australis* departed, carrying the Davis and Mawson crew along with ten Chinese expeditioners to be dropped off at a Chinese base and twenty-one members of the Prince Charles Mountain Expedition program. From the deck, streamers linked families on the dock as a crew member slipped the line off the bollard. As the 'AA' pulled out, one girl in the crowd on the dock became hysterical, screaming for her dad, begging him not to go, not to leave her. Streamers broke around her, the ends fluttering down as she continued to cry. It was gut-wrenching to watch.

The expeditioners handled the departure in a variety of ways. A few subtly wiped their eyes. My stomach was hollow, filled only with homesickness. This second departure was harder than the first to Macca.

The motion of the ship was constant as the 'AA' fought with the waves of one of the world's unfriendliest oceans. The Circumpolar Current is driven by some of the strongest winds on earth. Sailors call the southern latitudes the 'Roaring Forties', the 'Furious Fifties' and the 'Screaming Sixties', for good reason. Seasickness claimed me again. I was unable to leave my bunk for a couple days as I tried to cope with it. I could not hold any food down so our Davis doctor, Dr John Cadden , "Cad", gave me injections to counter dehydration.

On the 30th at 8am we saw our first iceberg. Word spread and everyone climbed out of their bunks and onto the deck with video cameras capturing the moment. The 'AA' started pushing through ice once we hit the ice pack with large chunks being broken and pushed aside. The voyage became more bearable with calm conditions although snow was falling. Icebergs started to become more common and looked like massive land masses in the distance. At night, the 'AA" would switch on its searchlight to help avoid large bergs.

On the 3rd December I joined all the expeditioners on the trawler deck for the traditional sixty degree "South Crossing the Antarctica Circle" initiation. All virgins, including me, who had never crossed the line were forced to front King Neptune (Geoff Fulton – Beacon – dressed up) and Queen Neptune (deputy voyage leader) and their two pirate helpers. One by one King Neptune would call us up, and the pirates forced us to kneel, pick up a rotten fish which we had to offer to the sky before kissing it. Then they smeared Vegemite through our hair and onto our faces, much to the cheers of the onlookers. Once we passed the initiation, King Neptune gave us a certificate proclaiming the feat of crossing the sixty-degree line.

I sat and watched everyone go through the initiation and wondered why the odd person quickly disappeared. I soon found out when I went back to my cabin for a shower and found there was no hot water.

Late the next day the 'AA' anchored off Zhong Shan, the Chinese base not far from Davis. The following morning the two helicopters from the 'AA' flew the Chinese expeditioners and supplies into the base.

After lunch, the 'AA' continued its voyage chewing through ice and arriving at Davis late afternoon. Repeatedly the 'AA" kept on ramming forward and reversing until it broke through the thick ice within a certain distance of the base, so the fuel hose lines could be connected from the ship to the bulk fuel farm tanks. With a final clang, the 'AA' stopped, surrounded by solid ice. There were coloured buildings in the distance – my home for the next year.

Davis station sits on the edge of the Vestfold Hills, one of the largest ice-free areas on the continent, an area of approximately 400 square kilometres of low hills broken by valleys, deep fjords and lakes. The hills isolate the station from the icy plateau and the Sørsdal Glacier.

I watched heavy vehicles inch their way across the strong thick ice to start transferring our gear and supplies to the base. The next morning, we all disembarked including the 21 members of the Prince Charles Mountain expedition who flew on by a Twin Otter to their destination.

> ***I disembarked from the 'AA' and stood on the solid sea ice in Prydz Bay. The scene was breathtaking with icebergs jutting out from the frozen distance. In the crisp air, I was gripped with a heady mix of exhilaration and isolation.***

Cathie, Beacon and I walked the kilometre to the dark blue Met building where we met the outgoing crew members. The next few days I worked at the Met office learning my new role.

Part of the daily routine was the release of two weather balloons. Each one carried aloft a radiosonde that transmitted back temperature, air pressure, humidity, wind speed and direction as it ascended through the atmosphere.

Unlike the anxiety I had felt at Macca, learning the new routine at Davis was a straightforward and relaxed curve.

The outgoing Station Leader officially welcomed us, told us the station rules and advised us not to be stressed by all the activity. There were tents everywhere and beds set up army-style in any available space. All up there were about seventy people during the summer season and this overlap period stretched accommodation and the mess at mealtimes to the limit.

The re-supply period was chaotic with everyone working long hours. I was duelling with the person I was replacing from 5.15am until 10.15pm.

At night I was sleeping on a mattress on the floor in a room at the yellow Communication building. My permanent room would not be available until the old crew left.

I was having trouble sleeping. The glare from outside was unbelievable. We had to pull down the blinds to try to make some darkness. With the 24-hour summer sunlight my brain was not handling the continuous sunshine. I knew my body would take some time to get used to the unnatural 24-hours of daylight. It felt like a never-ending day.

After four days, the tractors and trucks stopped travelling the sea ice highway and the resupply had completed. After handshakes and toasts, we gathered at the edge of the sea ice holding red smoke flares in Antarctica tradition and said our final goodbyes to the old crew as the 'AA' departed for Mawson.

Once the old crew left, I finally got access to my room. I spent hours cleaning as the previous tenant had no time to do any cleaning before leaving. I was lucky to have a room on the coast side, with a brilliant view of the Islands and the sea from my window.

Jeremy approached me a few days before Christmas, offering me a jolly (a pleasure trip away from work). He required a team of three to go by chopper to collect pure virgin ice from the plateau for our upcoming Christmas and New Year's drinks.

I had no hesitation in saying yes. My stomach tightened as I approached the chopper, determined I could do this. I climbed in behind the pilot and focused on drawing deep breaths to slow my racing heart. My panic and anxiety disappeared as the chopper gained height.

A moonscape is the nearest description of the area surrounding our home: there was no vegetation, just dry, endless expanse of black rocks and cliffs. The chopper headed inland towards the plateau, over turquoise crystal-clear lakes dotted through the rocks. We crossed onto the Continental Ice Plateau with thousands of massive blue fingers of deep crevasses as far as we could see.

Gradually the crevasses became fissures, then solid ice where the pilot set us down. We were concerned with an approaching storm, so we only had a short time to break the ice into small blocks with a chainsaw, picks and crowbars.

It was hard, frustrating work trying to pry out the ice especially when I had to carry the large blocks back to the chopper.

The pilot pointed to the sky, "Come on, time to wrap this up. It's too dangerous to stay."

We were about 10 minutes ahead of the storm front as the chopper, full of ice, crossed back over the crevasses and left the plateau behind, heading for the moon-like rocks of Vestfold Hills and to Davis.

Christmas morning greeted us with the stark black rocks outside lightly hidden by falling snow. I rang Deb and the kids, and listened to their plans for the day.

As always on special occasions while far away from them, my feelings of homesickness intensified.

During the morning, the Davis Choir sang a range of Christmas carols before Santa's procession arrived on quad bikes. Many of us, including me, received packages from home. Families had been able to secretly mail packages marked "Christmas", to ANARE and it was arranged for them to come on the 'AA'. The meal, prepared by Gerbil and summer chef, Meredith, was again outstanding. I enjoyed the meal immensely, but I could not relax as I had to work in the evening at the Met office.

After Christmas I came down with the dreaded Davis flu, a particularly nasty strain of flu that had arrived with us on the 'AA' and gradually spread throughout the station. I watched everyone else come down with it and thought I had managed to avoid it, but it finally caught up with me. My throat was red raw, and there were headaches, a runny nose and painful coughs. I missed the New Year's celebrations, done in Davis-style with a 'D' Theme Party.

> *I did manage to haul myself down to the mess as 'D' for Dave shortly before midnight to cheer in the count of the New Year before leaving the fun behind and crawling back into bed..*

Mid-January, the sea ice had melted far enough to leave clear water to the islands a few kilometres away, allowing boating activities to start. Each calm day or evening, zodiac boat trips were organised, some for work purposes and others just for fun. One sunny and clear evening I managed to get on one of the two zodiacs for an iceberg tour to photograph icebergs and penguins.

We left the station's shore rugged up against the cold. For several hours we weaved around huge icebergs keeping our distance as the well-known expression "just the tip of the iceberg" took on a realistic meaning. Icebergs are inherently unstable and can collapse into many pieces, creating large waves. As we passed through ice floes, penguins stood on their ice rafts watching us go by. We passed a tabular berg – an iceberg with a flat top and sheer sides. The jagged peaks and ice caves caught my imagination the most. We slowed beside one iceberg with two green peaks, the unusual colour caused by organisms captured within the ice layers. The green really stood out against the stark whiteness of other icebergs and the blue of the ocean. As we manoeuvred by yet another iceberg, I was filming with my video camera when we heard a dreaded loud crack. It was just what we been trying to avoid, and Jeremy, the Station leader, immediately floored the engine of the zodiac to escape. The other expeditioner and I flew backwards into the bottom of the zodiac with my sunglasses flying into the ocean. We paused a safe distance away, engines idling, and waited and waited. It refused to roll. We finally had to give up and leave, back to the station.

Mid-month, I had to pass a 14.25 kilometres navigation walk through the Vestfold Hills as part of my field training. A group of us led by trainer Psycho (he was with me at Macca), set off at 9am from the base and we had to navigate using a compass and local terrain to Lake Dingle and back. I started strongly but it was not long before blisters formed. I kept shifting my full pack load as I negotiated the rocks, pebbles and steep hills, and eventually I pulled the same calf muscle that I had injured at Macca. Another expeditioner also pulled a muscle and the two of us struggled behind the main group. We finally arrived back at the station at 3pm, about 20 minutes after the main group, sore and tired but successful in all our tests.

At the end of the month it was my turn to go and learn field survival, navigation, quad driving, snow climbing, crevasse rescue and first aid training. Once again Psycho was our field training officer and I was joined on the field training by Jim (carpenter), Curtis (electrician), Dave (electrician) and Matthew (summer photographer).

I took a deep breath and climbed into the chopper. We lifted off, and once again I looked in awe at the landscape below with rich deep-blue lakes dotted among the dark rocks standing out against the sheer white of the ice plateau. After twenty minutes we were at our destination at Trajer Ridge base camp on the edge of the ice plateau.

The training equipment was waiting for us, having been brought out in the first days of the summer season slung below helicopters. After setting up our tents our first training exercise was to ride quads (Honda TRX300s), four-wheel drive cycles fitted with high-flotation tyres powered by a four-stroke petrol 300cc single cylinder engine. Quads were our main transport at and around the station, so we had to get used to them.

We left the base camp for the ice plateau and Psycho pointed out different features we had to keep an eye out for such as potholes, clear ice, crevasses and thin ice. Clear ice was our biggest worry. The quads lost all grip on it. If we were unlucky enough to hit a patch, we had to know how to get ourselves out of the situation. Learning to travel over different terrain angles was a tense experience until we learned to compensate for the various angles with our bodies and bums on the seat, backwards, forwards and sideways.

On arrival at Platcha Hut, we did a radio check to the main base, debriefed what we learnt and had a hot cuppa tea. After we had warmed up, Psycho got us to do ice cliff climbs to learn snow and ice techniques. These were gruelling as every movement had to be controlled and gradual. A few hours later, exhausted and cold, we climbed back onto the quads and headed to Sprunky's van where we would be spending the night.

On our way we were in dangerous territory with some thin patches of ice around. I was following Jim when we heard a crack, the ice split and I jarred to a stop, sitting in water to my knees. Curtis, who was behind me pulled up in time, climbed off his bike and threw a rope to me. I tied it on to my bike and his quad pulled me out. We could see the others in the distance waiting for us to catch up, but we decided to take a longer route around the thin ice to join them. When we caught up, Psycho said it was a good introduction to the afternoon lessons and showed us all how to get quads out, driving his into a thin patch. Working as a team, he showed us how to use ropes, spikes and picks to get the quad back out. We spent the rest of the afternoon and evening practising getting quads and people out of broken ice.

When we finished and arrived at Sprunky's van, it was time to cook a meal and get our bivvy bags ready. Psycho would be staying in the van, but the rest of us had to find ourselves some protection from the wind and bury ourselves in our bags.

It was light as the sun would only disappear below the horizon for about thirty seconds before rising again but the Katabatic winds coming from the plateau were blowing thirty plus knots, and I knew it would be a long night. It was. Not only was it bloody cold and windy, it was uncomfortable breathing in the confined space. The moisture from my breath froze, and icicles formed inside the bivvy bag.

> ***Once again, I struggled with claustrophobia and had flashbacks of me trapped in my pit hole back in Vietnam.***

The next morning, I was stiff from sleeping on the rocky ground. Psycho made us porridge for breakfast before we loaded our gear on the quads and headed back for Trajer Ridge. We continued our training, including self-saving while sliding down snow and ice, rope work and navigation. In the afternoon we practised rope work, descending into small crevasses and learning how to climb out. That night I shared a tent with Jim, who snored like a chainsaw.

I tied a rope around my ankle to the sleeping bag to prevent me escaping the tent in case of a nightmare.

The next day, our final training day, we put a quad over an ice cliff and used pulleys and ropes to get it back up. After lunch, our final session was abseiling over an ice cliff. One by one we took turns stepping off the edge and lowering ourselves down the cliff and back up.

We were finished. We packed our gear and gathered at a distance and watched the helicopters slingload the quads and transport our gear back to Davis. Our group were the last to leave Trajer Ridge by helicopter to the station.

In the first week of February we had our first medical emergency. The station received a call from a nearby Chinese ship, where one of the crew had fallen and suffered suspected broken ribs. He was brought in by a Chinese helicopter and rushed to our medical building, where Jim and I scrubbed up to help Dr Cad with X-rays. Dr Cad cleared him of any severe medical condition and diagnosed him with only bruising. He was given tablets and flown back by chopper to his ship.

With the return of the Prince Charles Mountain expeditioners, the station had again swelled to its limits. There were ninety-six expeditioners at Davis and no accommodation room available, so a lot of the expeditioners had to sleep in tents.

The '*Polar Bird*' arrived on the 7th February, an indication the summer program was near the end. The barge from the ship brought in fresh fruit and vegetables and mail.

After three days with all the empty fuel drums, recycled materials plus rubbish loaded along with the summer scientists, the '*Polar Bird*' sounded her horn and departed. We farewelled the ship in traditional Antarctica style with red flares. This left fifty-four of us at the station. Suddenly there was room everywhere – at the mess tables, in the laundry and for showers.

It was beginning to feel like heaven for me.

The morning before the first Ozone-Sonde launch, the Chinese ship '*Xue Long*' anchored in the bay and we hosted several Chinese expeditioners through the Met office.

The Met team of Cathie, Beacon and I, along with Tony who was with the Light Detection And Ranging program (LIDAR) launched the first Ozone-Sonde on the 21st February. We were taking part in the inaugural program of stratospheric ozone studies which had been established at Davis by the Australian Antarctic Division's Space and Atmospheric Sciences (SAS) group and the BoM. This was the first time that Australia was making in-situ measurements of stratospheric ozone in Antarctica and was part of a larger investigation at Davis by the SAS program to investigate the composition, dynamics and climate of the middle atmosphere. The Ozone-Sondes would be released monthly, increasing to weekly from mid-June to mid-October.

Near the end of the month, Jeremy asked me if I wanted to go to Zhong Shan, the Chinese base in the Larsemann Hills (120 kilometres from Davis). Besides the Chinese station, there was Progress 2 (Russian) and Druzhnaya 'A' (Russian summer-only-base) in the area at the east edge of the Amery Ice Shelf.

Courtesy visits were made to all these stations to re-establish friendly contact and to offer any help needed in the future. Jeremy thought it would be a good chance for me to take a trip there, especially as I spoke to the Chinese Met officers daily by radio to obtain their weather observations. For me this was a chance to see different parts of Antarctica.

A group of six including me were split into two groups for the trip on two helicopters. The timing had to be right to do such a trip with blue skies and little cloud as helicopters were not allowed to fly in heavy overcast skies in Antarctica for fear of whiteout. We took off and passed the icefalls and crevasses on the edge of the ice plateau. On the way we had to land to repair two all-weather stations (AWS) damaged by strong winds. At the first, as the repairs went on, I huddled against the bitter cold which was about -40°C with the wind chill factor. A group of four including me had to hold a tarp over the technician to protect him from the freezing wind so he could repair the AWS.

> ***I was overwhelmed with the isolation. I kept wriggling my toes and stamping my feet. As I breathed against the wind, the condensation of my breath froze until I had icicles hanging from my nose and moustache.***

At the second AWS, 60 kilometres away, the technician had to climb to the top of a mast pole to repair a wind-speed probe instrument. Snow was drifting and the wind was howling, making talking difficult. When finished, we flew to the coast with its sheer icebergs, ice cliffs and ice caves. The scenery was much more spectacular than around our station.

The Zhong Shan base was new with all modern amenities. We were greeted by the station leader. The officer-in charge of their Met program, Xu Cong, acted as our translator. My only Chinese was limited to hello and goodbye, which I put to good use as I greeted Xu's fellow Met workers, Lu Fei and Wan Jun – neither could speak English. After tea and biscuits, Xu took us on a tour of the station and then onto their Met office. He was especially proud of their new accommodation block. I spent about an hour-and-a-half comparing instruments and the set-up. After a gift exchange of bottles of spirits, I headed down the hill to the Russian station 'Progress', about a kilometre away where the others and the choppers were waiting for me. The Russian base was an eyesore … no other way to describe it. Rusting junk was piled up everywhere, with old fridges in one area, old tractors and machinery in another. With all the emphasis on protecting the environment, I could not believe the station looked so dreadfully untidy.

After catching up with my group, the Russian doctor offered to show us around his surgery which our doctor Cad eagerly accepted. The Russian doctor proudly pointed out various bits of equipment dating back to the 1950s. Cad was amazed at how far outdated their equipment was compared to ours.

I soon found out why there was so much tension as the only Russian to welcome us was the doctor. On a previous visit by the Australians, apparently the Aussies managed to drink quite a bit of their good vodka leaving them almost dry and wore out their welcome. When we lifted off about twenty Russians appeared waving us goodbye.

The trip back to Davis was spectacular. Our pilot flew low

along the coast to show us the crevasses and caves, with huge jagged walls of white towering above the ocean.

Although I still felt apprehensive about getting into choppers, I was becoming more comfortable within myself after the number of trips I had at Davis.

On the 2nd March, the *Aurora Australis* anchored near the shore at 7.30am and this was the official end of the summer season. Before the departure we farewelled the summer expeditioners and the two helicopters at the helipad and then made our way down to the shore.

At 2pm we lit red hand-held flares and cheered as the 'AA' sounded its horn and pulled out. It was the beginning of the winter season and she was the last ship to visit Davis until November.

It was an eerie feeling as I watched the ship disappear in the distance. My feelings were slightly dampened with the worry of my family as there was no way out for at least eight months.

There was an immediate difference in the station with only twenty-four of us left wintering. We all soon established our daily routine. In between shifts, I found a chance to practise my new-found hairdressing skills. Jim and I gave each other haircuts with clippers, putting our training to good use. I started getting customers but the females went elsewhere!

For hydroponics, other team members and I had to start from scratch by pulling out the old set-up and planting new seedlings of lettuce, tomatoes, cucumbers, snow peas, chillies (a favourite for our chilli beer), basil, parsley, sage, bok choy, zucchini, eggplant, celery, spinach, capsicum and shallots. After a while, we were rewarded for our hard work in the hydroponics shed with fresh salads and freshly cooked vegetables on the dining table at night. My turn in the hydroponics shed was on Thursdays. It was a welcome relief from the harsh outdoors with no vegetation around. As soon as I entered and took in the warmth and the smells, I happily shut the outside behind me and occupied myself in a pleasant way tending to the delicate growing plants.

The bright lights, greenery and warm moist atmosphere made me feel relaxed, free from tension and anxiety.

I was also a member of the home brew club brewing various batches of beer. I only attended once a fortnight because of shift work. For the fire team I was an acting BA Controller-breathing apparatus control officer who streamlined the calculations and monitoring of air usage and times for the fire team.

For entertainment we continued the traditional Friday night drinks with an informal meal, and we dressed up for formal Saturday night dinners, complete with tablecloths and candles. Every Tuesday night I joined a group in the green store for Volley Gin, a friendly game of volleyball followed by gins at the bar. We also had outdoor activities like the Davis Fishing Competition – Antarctica Style where each contestant had a drilled hole in the sea ice to fish from. Another big day was the Golf day on a five hole ice fairway.

A couple days before Anzac Day (April 25), Jeremy asked me to read the 'Ode to the Fallen' as I was the only veteran on the station. I was unsure at first as I had bad memories from previous Anzac days but in the end, I said "yes" as I felt it was my duty and I did not want to let my fellow expeditioners down.

I struggled with my thoughts before I could answer "yes".

On Anzac Day we gathered outside the comms building near the flagpoles at 10am for the dawn service. The flag was lowered to half-mast with snow falling lightly. Jeremy said a few words of introduction before I read the Ode. Tony played the Last Post on his trumpet and a minute's complete silence was then followed by the flag being fully raised to the masthead. After the ceremony we moved back into the warmth of the mess and played a traditional game of two-up with Anzac biscuits and drinks.

It ended up being more personal than I thought. I felt warmth and respect from the other expeditioners. I felt it was the first time since I returned from Vietnam that I had been accepted and acknowledged for my service to my country. Back in Australia we Vietnam veterans were ignored and humiliated for serving our country.

By the end of April, the sea ice was thick enough in most places for quads to travel on. Finally, on the 11th May around midday I was able to go on my first jolly on a quad with Gil (Mechanic) and Mark (Optical Physicist). It was overcast and about -20°C. Excited to leave the base to explore the surrounds we headed north on the sea ice, keeping the coast on our right and passing by Flutter and Lake Islands before turning into the coast towards Law Cairn about five kilometres from the base. We found the cairn packed under rocks. A tin box contained copies of historic documents at the site of the flag-raising ceremony conducted by Philip Law in 1954. It was the first ANARE landing in the area and an important precursor to the establishment of an Australian presence. After signing a registered visitor's book, we headed to Brookes Hut in Shirokaya Bay for a short break and a cup a tea.

After the break we continued towards Bandit's Hut. We made steady progress with Mark manning the GPS (Global Positioning System-navigation device) while Gil and I used the map. The only visible colours besides our bright clothes were white, blue and black. It was a good day to travel on the quads, but the motorised speed really intensified the wind chill factor. We followed the GPS and map northeast past Soldat and Partizan Islands before turning east into Long Fjord. We found Pioneer Crossing before moving north into Tyrne Fjord and we arrived at Bandit's Hut at 3pm. Established in 1983 on the north-west side of Tryne Fjord to support seal research, it is the furthest spot away from Davis about 26 kilometres north-east and can only be accessed via sea ice or helicopter.

Once inside Bandit's hut, we immediately got the gas heater and stove going to counter the damp cold. In the evening we relaxed and sat down to have Gerbil's stew and rice, a few gins and Baileys, played cards and then into our sleeping bags for a good night's sleep.

The next morning around 10.30am, I filmed the sunrise from the hut looking towards Barrier Island with spectacular views of the pristine surface of sea ice. After we fuelled our quads, we headed north past Mikkelsen's Cairn on one of the last islands in Prydz Bay, before turning back along the northern edge of the Vestfold Hills and on to Sir Hubert Wilkins Cairn in Walkabout

Rocks. It was here that Sir Hubert took possession of the area for England, and left a cairn with a flag and a copy of the declaration at the site. We climbed the steep hill and studied the spot before signing the visitor's book. It was a good opportunity to practise ice stops sliding down the hill.

Our plan was to return to Davis via the coastal route through the icebergs, but we kept encountering rafted ice (sheets of sea-ice piled one against the other) so opted to head back via Tryne Sound. Along the way we stopped to drill into the ice and measure the thickness (even jollies have duties). We followed a GPS route which took us out into Prydz Bay. The snow was thick with heavy drifts and areas of rafted ice, but Mark led us out when he found a clear route. In the afternoon we stopped at Rookery Lake Apple, about halfway back to Davis, for a cuppa and lunch. Mark was complaining about his feet, something we were wary of because of the danger of frostbite. After a rest, we separated, Gil headed back to Davis while Mark and I took the scenic iceberg route home. We made good time on the smooth ice but slowed at times on rafted ice. We got back to the station in fading daylight at about 4.45pm. When I took my helmet off the look of horror on Mark's face told me something was wrong. I felt a fist-sized lump below my chin and knew it was frostbite. It had swelled out of my chin, neck area and was seeping blood, forcing me to visit Dr Cad.

The frostbite happened after we left Rookery Lake Apple when I put my helmet on and it pushed my neck warmer down, allowing air to flow below my helmet and under my chin. I should have been wearing a balaclava like Mark and Gil for protection but was only wearing a neck warmer and beanie.

CHAPTER 25

Dr Cad treated the frostbite and warned me that I would need treatment for at least several weeks. I ended up with a small scar on my chin, the size of a five-cent coin. I expected some pain but did not feel any. After the experience, Jeremy issued me with a balaclava.

In my spare time I volunteered to help other expeditioners with their duties, the sea ice observation team, the biologist team of Chad and Nanette and the Science team of Malcom and Paula.

For the sea ice observation, we headed by quads to various established spots marked by bamboo canes up to six kilometres offshore, to drill through and measure ice thickness and snow cover. The measurements served two purposes: whether the ice can support people and equipment and be part of a long-term glaciological research program.

Biologists Chad and Nanette were studying viruses in the saline lakes of Ace, Pendant and Highway Lakes for concentrations of micro-organisms. Viruses were common in the lakes and were threatening the bacteria and phytoplankton (single-cell organisms which form the basis of the marine food chain and play a key role in the exchange of carbon dioxide between the atmosphere and ocean).

We headed north to Long Peninsula, where all three lakes were located. Our quads were loaded up with gear, which we had to man-pack over heavy rocks to get to the different lakes. Once at a lake, Chad and Nanette unpacked before drilling through the thick surface to take water temperatures, radiation readings and water samples at various depths. The water was then deposited into sample containers and taken back to the station to be checked by a microscope for organisms.

Scientists, Malcolm and Paula, worked on Crooked Lake deploying remote environmental monitoring equipment. They always needed help setting up their equipment.

> ***Helping the different teams gave me a sense of satisfaction and was a chance for me to check out icebergs and the surrounding areas near Davis. I was overwhelmed by the beauty.***

The 2nd of June was the last day the sun would rise above the horizon for a while. It stayed above from 1320 to 1411 hours, a final gift of 51 minutes of sunshine. Midwinter is often blamed for problems like sleep disorders, depression and conflict between expeditioners.

In our group, everyone handled the experience differently. Some chose to spend their downtime in their rooms, while others focussed on indoor activities like watching different movies in the comfortable seats of our movie theatre.

> ***I took the opportunity to take guitar lessons from Tony (Physicist) and completed my Hagglunds theory-practical driving test.***

Hagglunds is a Swedish made dual-cab-over-snow vehicle equipped to carry four people in the front cab while the rear cab can be used for gear and equipment. They can travel over most terrain, including sea ice and soft snow, and have a range of 250 kilometres.

Gil put me through my lessons on handling and driving the vehicle including steering, revs over different terrain and reversing. Reversing between bamboo sticks was by far the hardest to learn. I had to concentrate on the back section, using the mirrors to manoeuvre between the bamboo sticks but after a few attempts I managed to finally get through.

Gil was satisfied and I passed both my theory and practical.

It was Mid-winter 21st June, the biggest date on the Antarctica calendar. Not only is it the winter solstice, it is also the approximate mid-point of the expedition and the celebration is a tradition going back to Scott's first Antarctic expedition in 1901.

Activities started early with a chicken and champagne breakfast, followed by successive dips in cold and hot spas. It was traditional to swim in a hole in the sea ice, but this year they had not been able to make a big enough hole. They used explosives to break through, but the chainsaw failed when they tried to enlarge the hole.

A few of the younger expeditioners were disappointed but I was never going to get in myself as Dr Cad warned a few of the older expeditioners including me of the dangers of the shock causing heart problems.

Plumbers, Paul and Cal, built an outdoor cold spa and an indoor hot one in the tank room. Throughout the day we took turns sipping on champagne and relaxing in the hot water. Late in the afternoon we gathered in the mess for the lavish feast prepared by Gerbil. Every place setting had a decorated menu featuring photos of all of us. Once we sat down, Jeremy (Station Leader) took the floor and welcomed everybody to the celebration and read out some of the fifty messages Davis received including those from politicians and other Antarctica Stations. Then we started the feast, a range of all sorts of food, so substantial that one buffet was barely touched.

Entertainment followed with about ten expeditioners taking to the stage for the pantomime 'Jack and the Beanstalk' (with an ANARE slant) to entertain us. The group left us in stitches, especially with the veiled ANARE twists to the much-loved old storyline.

The sun finally made an appearance on the 11th July after thirty-eight days below the horizon. Our first official day of sunshine from 1331 to 1416 hours.

We were now able to leave the station and explore the surrounds.

On the 3rd August, Mark, Tony, Gil and I left for Watts hut after lunch. The temperature was minus seventeen degrees Celsius and there was light snow. We travelled on the sea ice and halfway along Ellis Fjord our quads started struggling to keep their grip on the blue ice. I had to find the correct balance of power on my quad to prevent skidding sideways. Fortunately, the hut was not far and the whole trip took about half an hour.

The view was magnificent, a gentle landscape with the long seemingly smooth fjord behind. The red hut was nestled in between the north eastern shore of Watts Lake and Ellis Fjord. We explored the surrounds, but I discovered my camera did not work due to the freezing conditions.

From then on, I put all my camera gear inside my yellow freezer suit between my singlet and thermal gear.

We spent the rest of the night in the cosy hut and after dinner we played poker. The next day at 11.30am we headed towards Trajer Ridge and the ice plateau where we did our field training. We had a clean run until we came to narrow ridges, some with massive drop-offs. To cross the ridges, I would have to put my weight on the quad on the side opposite the drop-offs and take it slow.

It was nerve-wracking and I had to concentrate hard.

From Trajer Ridge we went onto the ice plateau and followed the edge of the plateau to Sprunky's Van, where we had bivvied for the night during the summer training. We wanted a last look at the van, which was scheduled to be moved back to Davis permanently.

On our way back to Watts hut just past Trajer Ridge melon, Tony pulled up sharply and we followed. Cautiously we got off the quads and went to see what was wrong. A massive four-foot wide crevasse had split the ground. In shock, we studied it, looking down into the seemingly endless depth. We had travelled over this exact spot on the way to Sprunky's Van and the ice had obviously collapsed behind us and I realised I was the last in the line at the time.

It was a reminder that nothing is certain out there. We were living and working in a fragile environment. What seemed solid and stable could change in a minute.

Subdued, we skirted right around the area back to Watt's Hut, with our headlights cutting our path on the last stretch.

Morning came quickly. We cleaned up, loaded the black box (for our toilet solids) onto the back of one of the quads and left at 11.30am for Crooked Lake. There we met up with Cal, Cad and Beacon who were helping Malcolm with his research on the lake. After catching up, we headed to the east side of the lake to climb Boulder Hill, a ten-minute trek which offered superb views.

Our goal was to get to Sørsdal Glacier, which is accessed by the far western side of Crooked Lake, by the frozen rapids at Mossel Lake and Chelnok Lake, but we could not find the path. It was clear on the map, but we could not get across the ridges. We missed the narrow entry several times as we went up and down the area. Finally, the gap revealed itself and we made our way to the glacier. When we arrived, it was heavily overcast, and we could not make out the line between the glacier and the sky or see its true colours.

It was disappointing as others had raved about this massive slow-moving glacier. Even so, we walked along the glacier for a while and wondered what it would look like in clear weather. The Sørsdal is one of the key polar outlet glaciers that contribute to the drainage of the East Antarctic ice sheet. Then it was time to head back, via Watts Hut (to pick up the rest of our gear and rubbish), back along Ellis Fjord to Davis at 5pm.

It had been an exhilarating few days especially after the scares with the crevasse and drop-offs.

The 11th August was a new low for us when the temperature reached a low of minus 32.1 degrees Celsius. I did not think it could get any colder, but it did on the 13th August when it got down to minus 32.7 degrees Celsius. I stayed indoors as often I could with these conditions but work required me to venture out to take weather readings. I was always concerned with blizzards.

I would lie in bed at night and listen to the strong gale force winds which sounded like a roaring train passing by outside. I dreaded and feared the walks in the dark from the accommodation building to the Met office in those blizzard conditions. I experienced six blizzards while at Davis with wind gusts over 70 knots (129.6 km/hr), the highest wind gust at 76 knots (140.7 km/hr) on the 30th August.

When I headed out in blizzard conditions, I let either Cathie or Beacon know. I crawled along a rigging line permanently connected between buildings. I gripped onto the rope and forced myself forward through the limited white-out visibility. I was worried about any loose objects that could be lying around and become deadly missiles. With the pressure of the thick snow pushing into me, I could hardly breathe and kept gasping to get air into my aching lungs. I inched my way forward into the fury of the wind, relieved to reach each building along the way and I was very much relieved when I finally made it to the Met office.

Mentally my feelings were like when I came under fire from the Viet Cong in Vietnam but in Antarctica blizzard conditions the enemy was Mother Nature. On all these occasions adrenalin had consumed me, a fear of dying with my heart pounding as I reacted to the dangers.

With the approaching summer program, our cook, Gerbil, had progressively resupplied the various huts around the area, bringing back accumulated old food items to be sorted, eaten or burnt.

I went with Gil and Gerbil on the 20th August in a Hagglunds to the Rookery Lake Apple and to the Magnetic Island Melon to resupply new food. After we swapped the supplies of food at Rookery Lake, we then travelled through Iceberg Alley towards Magnetic Island taking photos of the more impressive arched bergs. The sun was out, making the entire landscape sparkle. We stopped to watch a solitary Emperor Penguin on the ice. We were puzzled as it was a long way away from the edge of the sea ice. At Magnetic Island again we sorted through the old food replacing it with new food. From there, I drove the Hagglunds the remaining five kilometres back to Davis.

I escaped the station confines again on the 26th for another jolly with Mark to check out icebergs in Iceberg Alley. We left Davis at around 12.30pm on quads in perfect conditions with temperature minus 22 degrees Celsius. Our targets were the spectacular jade and arched bergs and the trip did not disappoint. Neither did the emerging wildlife as we watched and were mesmerised by two Weddell seals in a water hole. On the way back to Davis in the late afternoon, Mark accidentally went into a snowdrift and bogged his quad. I tried to pull him out, but my quad got bogged too in the soft snow. It took us about forty-five minutes to dig and free both quads. We arrived back at Davis after 6pm.

> ***Whenever anyone left the station to go into the field, they had to turn their name tags over on the wall and let the Station Leader know where they were going. You also had to carry a quad tool emergency kit, first-aid kit, a shovel and a hand-held VHF radio.***

CHAPTER 25

Spring brings the best of Antarctica, with longer days, improving weather and still solid sea ice to travel on. We planned to use the period to get off the base to explore new areas and prepare for the upcoming summer program.

Large-scale planning started for two teams of expeditioners to go to the Rauer Group of islands, about 40 kilometres south of Davis. While not far, the route was unreliable and dangerous. To get there, we would have to go up to the ice plateau and across the glacier, avoiding crevasses along the way. For the upcoming summer program, a group of biologists would be working in the area investigating pollutants in sea birds. We were charged with checking the condition of the huts and stores. I was assigned to the second group leaving at the end of the month.

It was a sunny and clear morning on the 29th September at 7am, when a group of ten including me left Davis in two Hagglunds. We picked our way over snow and ice through the Vestfold Hills until we hit the Breid Basin at 8.40am, where we had to get out and walk up the steep ice ramp to put us on the plateau. The Hagglunds were loaded and pulling sleds, and for safety reasons we were not allowed to ride in them up the ramp in case they tipped over. It was hard work, taking us a good quarter of an hour to walk up the sharp gradient. We joined the Hagglunds at the top and followed the edge of the ice plateau south and two hours later we arrived at the old Russian fuel dump where rusted drums littered the pristine surface.

We continued, passing over plenty of slots on the Sørsdal Glacier and felt the Hagglunds as they dropped into the indentations. At 1.30pm, we came across something embedded in the ice. Neil (Mechanic) got out and peered at the object before calling us out. In the middle of thousands of square miles of empty ice was one of our Met radiosondes. We all climbed out and watched as Neil worked the ice pick to pry it out. "Bloody Morg," someone yelled out. "Polluting Antarctica with your balloons and radiosondes." I smiled as Neil held it up. It was like the proverbial needle in the haystack. According to the GPS, we were 24.6 kilometres from Davis. A few hours later, we reached Rauers ramp where we refuelled the Hagglunds. The first group had dropped off fuel supplies and quads for us. After we checked the decline of the ramp, I took over the driving and followed two of our group members on quads down the ramp from the ice plateau to the sea ice and continued to Hop Island.

There we unpacked and put up our tents before we headed to the nearby Melon on the island itself about fifty metres away to have dinner. We had covered 87.7 kilometres in five hours from Breid Basin.

I had nightmares often at new locations, and I knew I would feel claustrophobic in the tent.

Mark and I were sharing. In the cold porch area of the polar tent, I took off my boots and freezer suit leaving only my thermals on and crawled into the dry area where our bivvies and mattresses were.

I tied a cord around my ankle and attached it to the sleeping bag in case of a nightmare.

Once in my bivvy, I put on a dry pair of socks and tracksuit and curled up, but the chill found its way in. Like most of the others, I had a pee bottle with me and before sleep used it and tucked it down between my feet for warmth for a short time. (By morning, the pee bottle would be frozen.)

That night I only got broken sleep but no nightmares.

Next morning when we left the tent, we had blowing snow with 35 to 40 knot winds. After breakfast we headed to Filla Island hut, a short thirty-minute trip to drop off supplies and a gas bottle before continuing to Winterover Bay at the edge of the plateau. For the rest of the day, on our return trip back to camp via Sloan Island we searched for a piece of Australian history, a small aluminium canister containing records and flags left in the area somewhere by Sir Hubert Wilkins in 1939. Many expeditioners attempted to find the historic artefacts in the Rauer Islands area over the years, but none had been successful. We too had to admit defeat, leaving the area empty-handed and went back to camp. After a late meal and lively conversations in the Melon we headed to our tents for sleep with heavy snow falling.

The next day, our third, we headed to Macey Peninsula to drop off a food box and a drum of fuel as an emergency stash for future expeditions. The trip was difficult as there was no visual definition between the ground and the sky and there were several large drop-offs. Several of us including me had to get out, attach ourselves to the Hagglunds and guide them through the difficult areas.

Our fourth day was reserved for sightseeing around the Rauer Group of islands. We explored the stunning jade bergs and ice cliffs while still looking for that elusive canister. The jade bergs took on surreal qualities. One looked like the cartoon character Snoopy dog and another resembled a castle at Disneyland. Unfortunately, the weather started to deteriorate so we headed back to camp and by late afternoon we were in blizzard conditions. A call to Davis confirmed our worries that the blizzard had set in and would become progressively worse.

The next day our return to Davis was cancelled due to those blizzard conditions. It gave us a rare chance for a lazy day. I slept most of the day, occasionally peering out of the tent to check the conditions. I ventured to the Melon hut in the evening and found Gerbil had baked scones. After we had eaten them we crawled back on the thick snow to our tents and into our cold but dry sleeping bags insulated by a blow-up mattress.

> ***I curled up tight in an attempt to preserve my body heat and cursed the freezing cold night. I never felt warm during the night. The only time my feet were warm was when I peed in my bottle and pushed it to the bottom of the sleeping bag, but this only lasted about 15 minutes.***
>
> ***The howling wind had changed from an exciting reminder of our adventure to an ugly fear-inducing threat. During the long night I feared the tent would not survive its assault.***

We gathered in the morning to discuss options and I urged the group to take advantage of the break in the weather to head back to Davis. We radioed Beacon, who confirmed the satellite picture showed conditions improving. Gear was quickly stowed in the Hagglunds before we headed off at 8am. We arrived on the plateau via the Rauers ramp about ninety minutes later.

One of the Hagglunds had a broken coupling which forced us to leave one of the sleds loaded with fuel behind near the Rauers ramp but luckily the second Hagglunds was fine and we packed the quads onto the remaining sled. It was slow work as we had to rest for a few minutes behind the Hagglunds from the freezing forty-knots wind.

Finally, we headed back along the plateau until we hit the slotted and crevassed area of the Sørsdal Glacier. Two of our group members had get out and tied themselves to the Hagglunds to guide us cautiously through. We arrived back at Davis by 5pm.

I enjoyed my first shower in six days.

Activity back at the base continued to increase to finish the jobs before the arrival of the *Aurora Australis* with the new expeditioners and resupply. Every available space around the base was being prepared for summer accommodation.

On the 21st October we received a call that Dave P (Electrician) and Jeff (Carpenter) had been stranded on a hut maintenance trip. Their Hagglunds had overheated, forcing them to abandon it a couple of kilometres from Bandit's Hut where they spent the night. Early next morning Gil and I went out on quads to give them a hand. The wind chill meant we were riding into minus 50°C temperatures. Ten kilometres from Davis, we found the Hagglunds and Gil quickly found the problem, a coolant hose had exploded, and it did not take him long to replace it. Once the engine was running, we abandoned the quads and took the Hagglunds to Bandit's Hut to pick up the stranded expeditioners before returning to the quads. Gil and Dave P in the Hagglunds and Jeff and I on the quads returned to Davis via Iceberg Alley.

On the 25th October Gil started giving me Mack truck lessons. I had been selected to drive the truck to help with the resupply. My first driving mission was to carry an open container from the beach area to the nearby aerial farm in preparation for the resupply. In the evening of the same day, we had our final 'End of Winter Dinner'.

Our solitude officially ended on November 1st at 5pm, when three Canadians landed their fixed-wing Twin Otter on the sea ice outside Davis. They had left Calgary, Canada, and flown through America, South America and onto one of the American Antarctic bases before arriving at Davis. They were our first visitors in the eight months since March.

It signified that our close-knit group was no longer to be, with everyone keen to talk to them.

On the 3rd, the 'AA' left Hobart early in the evening for Davis.

Reality had set in that our winter was over and shortly I'd be preparing to pack up and leave.

Around this time the Bureau threw me a twist, asking if I would be interested in going to Casey for winter immediately after returning from Davis. I would be allowed a short break with my family before taking up the posting. They were desperate for an OIC for Casey as two previous successful candidates had withdrawn, and the Bureau had run out of time to find and train a replacement.

It was a hard decision. On the one hand I would finally get to Casey, which had always eluded me, and on the other hand, it was a big ask of my family especially after I have been away from them for fifteen months. I rang Deb to discuss the Casey job and she asked if I was serious. It was not an easy conversation. My family needed me and I agreed but another twelve months down on the ice would help to pay university fees and kitchen renovations that we had planned and the biggest plus would be not having to return to the Rockhampton office with staff in-fighting and dealing with the public.

Deb and the kids knew I would find it hard if I returned to work at Rockhampton with the long commutes to work and back so after discussing the pros and cons for the next few days, they agreed they could handle another year. I promised them I would retire after Casey. I rang the Bureau to let them know I would take the Casey OIC job.

On the afternoon of the 16th, we could see the 'AA' breaking through the sea ice as she approached Davis. She wedged into the ice about four kilometres from the station. Everyone came ashore and every available space at Davis was filled. The Twin Otter made several trips, taking the new winter crew into Mawson and bringing the old crew back to Davis so they could join us on the 'AA' back to Australia.

For the next three days, I was on truck duty, driving on the Sea Ice Highway, carrying waste from Davis to the 'AA' and returning with fresh supplies for the green store and fuel drums for the fuel farm. At times it was difficult to manoeuvre the big Mack truck, especially driving off the sea ice onto the beach area where the ice was breaking up under the constant traffic.

The resupply finished on the 19th and I started duelling with my replacement, showing him his duties in the Met office.

The formal changeover ceremony was held two days later, on the 21st, and Jeremy handed over the keys to the incoming station leader. We were all presented with our Antarctica medallions and then driven out to the 'AA' ready for the trip back to Fremantle via Zhong Shan. Just after 2pm, the 'AA' sounded the horn while the expeditioners on the ice set off flares, waving and dancing. As we started putting distance between us and the shore, I felt an immense sadness. My home for the past 12 months was fading into the distance. I had become attached to and shared my life with my fellow expeditioners. They were like family to me. This was the end of our time at Davis and the beginning of our new life journeys.

The 'AA' chewed through the ice, leaving chunks in her wake. At 8pm we got to within 18 nautical miles of Zhong Shan. The next morning the helicopters started the resupply of the Chinese base. I worked on the bridge doing weather reports for the helicopters. On the 23rd at 4.30pm, the resupply complete, we left Antarctica behind for Australia.

> ***On my journey back to Australia I had a routine outgoing psychological test, to find out how I had coped with the long period of remoteness. I felt I had coped very well and the isolation helped me find peace within myself although I was still having nightmares. My mask was strong and PTSD symptoms could be ignored in my new world of isolation.***

The following evening, we finally left the sea-ice pack and by the next afternoon the icebergs were gone. From there it got warmer by the day and on December the 3rd about 100 nautical miles off the Western Australian coast, I saw my first Australian bushfly for almost a year and I knew then I was nearly home.

The next morning, we were stationary between Rottnest Island and Perth, with the city's tall buildings and Scarborough Beach in the distance. We lined up among a dozen container ships waiting for a pilot. He climbed aboard at 1pm and an hour later we tied up at Fremantle wharf.

Saying goodbye was difficult. My feelings were mixed: the excitement of coming home but disappointment at leaving behind the beauty of the ice and the camaraderie. But reality was waiting. It was strange driving through the city; the heat, noise and traffic fumes were overwhelming and increased my anxiety.

I stayed the night with my older brother Gerry and his partner Rene and the next afternoon on the 5th December I caught a flight from Perth to Brisbane and then onto Rockhampton, arriving at 8.45pm where Deb, Michelle and David were waiting to greet me.

It felt good to touch them again and to see they were safe. My emotions were tight, I felt my heart was in two pieces – one here with my family and the other down south on the ice.

Culture shock with flies and dust had re-surfaced in my life. The musty earthy smell present after rain, and the odour of freshly cut grass assaulted my senses. It is the only way to describe returning to the mainland after almost a year in the spectacular, stark, sterile, forbidding Antarctica.

I knew I would have limited time with my family and wanted to make the most of it. The first few weeks at home was for family time and routine stuff like mowing lawns. Then we packed and headed off on a family holiday for several weeks in Caloundra, Brisbane, the Gold Coast and into New South Wales to Coffs Harbour and Port Macquarie. It was a peaceful time and I was lulled into holiday mode, enjoying the beach and relaxing.

I was starting to question my reasons for going back as it was enjoyable being home.

CHAPTER 26

CURSE OF CASEY BASE ANTARCTICA

When the clock finally ran out, I packed reluctantly and gave my family one last hug at the Rockhampton airport.

> ***It was never easy saying goodbye with anxiety, "butterflies" in my stomach and smothering feelings of unreality.***

In Hobart, I started the familiar training routine like how to order Met stores (weather balloons etc) by a new computer system model and attending fire training. This time I had been chosen for the 'Breathing Apparatus Team' at Casey, so I had to undertake a full fire training course, including entering a smoke-filled container to negotiate a course full of obstacles and rescue dummies at the Tasmania Fire Training Centre in Cambridge.

> ***Entering the smoke-filled container was difficult for me as my recurring nightmare was of me suffocating in the pit***

hole in Vietnam. Any closely confined space, darkness or any difficulty breathing caused extreme fear.

When I stepped inside the container filled with smoke my head was spinning with anxiety, but I forced myself to breathe air evenly from the regulator. I was in between two other fire trainees attached by rope, so not being alone helped. Fumbling in the dark with no sense of whereabouts, we eventually rescued the dummies.

I was told I could not get on the ship without a dental clearance so a visit to the dentist was next. Three fillings later, I was cleared and went back to the Antarctic Division in Kingston to be kitted out. My final duty before leaving was to report to Calvary Hospital for some tests. I needed some isotope imaging done. The stress test was done on a bike. I was injected with chemicals for the isotope imaging before pedalling like crazy. After 14 minutes on the hardest setting, I was medically cleared and ready to go.

After one week of training plus medicals, at 5pm on the 17th February, the 'AA' pulled away from the wharf amid farewell waves with its horn reverberating across the harbour.

My anxiety was high.

The next morning, I was up on the bridge early to do meteorological work but did not last long. As on previous voyages seasickness came upon me causing me to crawl into my bunk. I spent the next couple of days sliding from one end of my bunk to the other in heavy rough seas. With the ongoing seasickness the ship doctor visited to give me an injection to prevent dehydration.

I managed to get my strength back and by the time we reached and crossed the 60-degree line of initiation, I was up and about. I watched and cheered on the deck as King Neptune and his beautiful long-suffering Queen initiated the expeditioners crossing the line for the first time. That evening we had to put up with cold showers.

On February 24th we sighted our first iceberg, a majestic carved monument floating past us and early in the night we entered the sea-ice pack with weathered icebergs a regular occurrence.

On the morning of 26th February at 0630, we arrived at Casey. Shortly after I watched a LARC (lighter amphibious resupply cargo vessel) commence operations.

Staring at the coloured buildings, my home for the next eight months, I felt satisfied and relieved that I had finally made it to Casey on my third attempt and broken the curse of Casey. Now it was time to go ashore and meet her.

I climbed aboard the station work boat '*Pagadroma*' to take us ashore. After we docked, I walked to the Met office for the changeover procedures with the outgoing officer-in-charge (Cliff). After outlining my duties and showing me through the office, we went to the red shed (accommodation block) to inspect my room and have lunch.

I had been at Casey for just over three hours. I have no recollection of what happened next, but it was the beginning of a long nightmare. The following story of the accident, the medevac and voyage back to Australia was told to me by different expeditioners. I also read and got information from the daily Antarctic Division SITREP – Situation Reports.

After lunch, Cliff took me on a tour of the base and apparently at the edge of the base area we found ourselves on clear ice. We both slipped. Cliff saved himself while my head hit the ice. Cliff went for help and I was taken to the medical rooms in the red shed accommodation building. There were three doctors in attendance, the Casey doctor (Tanya), the 'AA' doctor (Jeff) and the ingoing Macquarie Island doctor (Andy). They diagnosed me with a severe head injury. They tried to take X-rays, but the scanned copies were not clear, so they contacted the Chief Neurosurgeon at the Hobart Hospital and discussed my medical condition. The decision was made to medevac me back to Australia as soon as possible.

Apparently, I came to that evening. I was in a high neck brace, connected to an oxygen mask and connected to drips. I rang Deb and the kids and had a brief conversation, telling them I arrived and had a fall and the doctors believed it was concussion. I would be ok and back at work in a couple of days' time.

> ***Deb later told me she thought something was wrong as I was speaking very slowly and was not making any sense. I have no recollection of the call.***

Dr Jeff got on the phone after I had finished and told Deb that in his medical opinion, "Dave should return home". He reassured her that I was coping and comfortable and promised to call with regular updates.

The next morning my condition did not improve. The neurosurgeon in Hobart was updated and told heavy blizzards had prevented the chopper from leaving the 'AA'. In the afternoon, the weather conditions improved. I was transferred from the bed to a stretcher, strapped in tightly to remain immobile and a bright orange plaid blanket tucked over me. The mood was sombre and about six expeditioners lifted the stretcher to their waist height, keeping me level as they descended the ramp outside the red shed with slow steps to the chopper. Snow was falling as they slid me in and strapped me down in the chopper with expeditioners gathered nearby shouting encouragement and various messages as the chopper lifted. Once on the 'AA', I was transferred to the hospital ward with drips attached to me.

> ***Just one day after I arrived at Casey, the 'AA' sounded its horn and departed at 7pm, leaving the 'Curse of Casey' behind.***

Doped up and full of painkillers, I spent the next five days in bed struggling against the pain in my head and neck with Doctors Jeff and Andy observing my condition. Dr Jeff contacted Deb every two days with updates on my condition. From the 4th March they slowly started to get me out of bed for short periods, putting me on a chair in the shower to wash me and on the loo to try and get my bowels working again. I tried eating something solid, rather than relying on drips. The first time I stood up, I nearly passed out due to the increased pressure in my head. Also, on the 4th March, Dr Jeff reminded me it was my birthday. They helped me to the mess to celebrate my birthday with a cake and the expeditioners sang "Happy 56th Birthday" to me.

> ***I simply could not appreciate it at the time as I struggled with the neck brace and the constant headache fogging my mind.***

The 'AA' dropped anchor in Buckles Bay, Macquarie Island on the 5th March at 7am. Cargo operations started a few hours later by LARC and chopper. Dr Jeff wanted me to be more mobile and helped me to the deck to watch the resupply.

It was the most I had walked in eight days and my head was spinning.

After two days the refuelling and cargo operations were completed. Dr Jeff decided it would be good rehabilitation for me to visit the solid ground on Macca so he arranged with the Voyage Leader for me to go ashore for a few hours. On the chopper we passed over the rugged coastline and circled over the old buildings before setting down. I went into the mess and rang my family, the first lucid conversation in a few weeks.

They were relieved to hear my voice. Deb was upset with the Bureau of Meteorology as they had not contacted her about my accident. Deb, Michelle and David were determined to meet me in Hobart when the ship arrived.

With Dr Andy's help I visited Garden Cove and the Met office before saying goodbye to Andy as he was about to start his 12-month stint on the Island. After three hours I returned to the 'AA' exhausted and with a splitting headache.

On the 9th, due to the forecast adverse weather conditions, all expeditioners were brought off Macca by lunchtime. The horn sounded at 2pm and I watched the flares being lit on a distant rock as the engines of the 'AA' started pulling us away.

I felt nothing, and certainly not the excitement or sorrow I usually had when seeing those flares.

We were travelling better than anticipated, evading the adverse weather conditions as forecast and we arrived in Hobart on the 12th March at 8am. As we approached the wharf, I started having mixed feelings, knowing it was likely to be my last trip on the *Aurora Australis* and my last expedition to Antarctica.

Dr Jeff helped me out to the deck where I searched the mass of faces for Deb, Michelle and David. I finally saw my family and I was not prepared for the strong emotions I felt when I finally hugged them. The crew of the 'AA' brought Deb, Michelle and David on board and gave them a tour, an unexpected bonus, and they got to see what it would be like to travel the Great Southern Ocean.

Before I left the 'AA' I met up with both Dr Gormly AAD and Dr Jeff and thanked them kindly, especially Jeff for taking care of me. They had arranged for me to be admitted to Hobart hospital to be treated for my head injury including an MRI scan (magnetic resonance imaging) to my head and X-rays to my neck later that afternoon.

I also met up with Beacon (ex-Davis), and BoM Chief Administrator Jenny who was very apologetic to Deb, realising that the Department had let the family down and told Deb to send all the receipts for the airfares and accommodation expenses to BoM to be reimbursed.

I had never had an MRI scan before and was unprepared for what was to come. At the hospital, they loaded me into the long tunnel which had a clearance above my head of perhaps 5cms. Strapping me in was bad enough but as I entered, I had a meltdown. Screaming, I was trapped in a full-blown anxiety attack and a flashback of being buried in the pit hole back in Vietnam.

They quickly pulled me out and I sat shaking, refusing to go back in. The next day they gave me some anxiety tablet to relax me before going in. Whatever the tablet was, it worked.

For the next eight days I was in and out of hospital for scans and X-rays while my head injury was monitored by a neurosurgeon. He told me I was a lucky boy and by rights I should not be alive. He believed that the cold freezing conditions had jelled the bleeding on the brain which saved my life. The scan pictures clearly showed the bruising of the brain. The neck X-rays showed ligament and muscle damage, especially down the left side where they had torn. It looked like I had subconsciously tried to keep my head up when I fell, causing the damage.

Clearly the doctors at Casey had made the correct decision to medevac me.

After three days touring Hobart and spending time with me, Deb, Michelle and David flew back to Yeppoon on the 15th. I had to wait for a clearance from the neurosurgeon to fly home due to the pressurisation of the aircraft cabin. During this period Beacon and his wife were my lifeline, driving me to doctors and physio appointments and reassuring me when I felt down. Another strong supporter was Dr Jeff, who checked on my progress every day.

On the 20th my neurosurgeon finally decided the bruising on my brain had reduced enough for me to fly and gave me the all-clear. To get on the flight to home, I had to sign a waiver to take full responsibility of my brain and neck injury.

This was the end of my Antarctica journey.

CHAPTER 27

MY REHABILITATION AND PTSD STRUGGLES AT HOME

For the coming months, I slowly started my rehabilitation at home. Worker's Compensation covered the time absent from work with weekly check-ups and physiotherapy. My head injury was progressing slowly but I suffered continuous headaches and dizziness. The neurosurgeon told me to expect a recovery period of 12-18 months.

My neck was also a problem. I was referred to a Pain Specialist in Rockhampton who injected cortisone into the C3, C4 and C5 vertebrae. Unfortunately, while it helped with the pain, I suffered a severe reaction, vomiting and breathing difficulties. Later, boils erupted all over my body.

For days I had dizzy spells and struggled to stay on my feet. My doctor checked my ears out and discovered a large hard blob of coagulated blood sitting on my left middle ear drum.

Apparently in the freezing conditions of Casey, the blood from my brain had coagulated after my head had hit the ice. I suppose no doctor had checked my ears.

This was a low period for me. Constant pain wears a person down, and I found I was in a deep hole of depression.

Coming back to Yeppoon I had a great deal of time on my hands. I had to accept that the Ice, a pivotal part of my life, was in my past. With my head and neck injuries, I would not be accepted for a posting down south again. For a long time, I struggled with the reality that my long-term goal and dream to work at Casey was over, rather like someone forced into retirement before he is ready. I had not chosen to leave but the choice had been made for me. Another sadness was the lack of loyalty by the Bureau, who failed to notify my family when I had the accident.

As I slowly healed, I went through different phases with my PTSD and depression. I had sad and negative beliefs about myself such as I am a failure, I am weak as I will never get over this head injury, I am cursed with the world against me and I have no future. I even had suicidal feelings. It was a bad period for me as I ended up in Yeppoon hospital with kidney stones and soon afterwards in Rockhampton hospital for 24 hours, for a ureteroscopy procedure. A laser was used to break up my small kidney stones.

After a lot convincing from Deb, Michelle and David, I started another phase of my life, I finally sought help for my **PTSD symptoms** that had haunted me for more than 40 years.

I was referred to Dr John Flanagan who started a long process of helping me to work through the after-effects of Vietnam-PTSD.

With ongoing counselling and psychological treatment with medication for PTSD, Dr Flanagan advised me I should not go back to work. I finally took notice and claimed for a disability pension at the special rate for Totally and Permanently Incapacitated (T&PI) through my local VVAA (Vietnam Veterans Association of Australia). My pension officer was a mate I had served with in Vietnam, Paddy Wilson who helped me to complete the forms and forwarded them to the Department of Veteran Affairs (DVA).

My claim for a full disability pension (T&PI) came through in early April 2005 and after this I retired from the Bureau of Meteorology on the 30th April 2005, after 33 years. It was the end of another era.

I had let go of my dream of isolation and now firmly set out on a path that would see me accept and deal with my PTSD demons. With continuing therapy treatment and counselling with Dr Flanagan my **nightmares**, which are my biggest problem, reduced in intensity and frequency from between seven to ten nightmares a week to three or four a week.

> ***I have two types of nightmares, one in which I scream and scramble out of bed in terror and the other, I am frozen and unable to get out of bed. With the first one, I am constantly afraid of seriously injuring myself while lost in the terror. In the past I had run into glass doors, walls and ended up with some shocking bruises.***
>
> ***My nightmares are triggered or exacerbated by things that***

prompt a reminder of my traumatic events. They can be as simple as noise, people or a reminder of places in Vietnam as well as my own personal feelings. The main triggers occur when I am tired, or I have been drinking alcohol. This is the reason I have not drank alcohol in recent times. During my nightmares I experience intense fear, helplessness and horror as I relive my trauma event.

Let me relate my nightmares 50 years on. Every night before I go to bed, I check all the doors are locked and windows closed. I unmake my bed, pulling the sheets and blankets out from all sides of the bed, something I have done since Vietnam. In my nightmares I am suffocating, cannot breathe, and feel as if I am dying with my body sweating profusely, moving and shaking in all directions before I jump out of bed screaming.

Any noise will set off my nightmares at night. It can be the sound of someone clicking a torch on and off, any house noises such as the flushing of the toilet, creaking of the house, and any noises from outside like dogs barking, car exhausts backfiring and sound of helicopters or planes flying nearby.

Catching up with veteran mates and drinking alcohol is another trigger causing distressing memories from the past. I try to avoid both, but it is hard, particularly on Anzac Day and Vietnam Veterans Day.

Any time when I go travelling to a new place and sleep in an unfamiliar bed in hotels or motels, I become unsettled and prone to nightmares.

With my **depression** I became so overwhelmed and sensitive over small issues that it led to aggressive **anger** outbursts. In mid-

2005 I got myself into a nasty altercation with a young chippie (builder) when he came into my property without permission to peg out surveyor points for a new house next door. I fronted him and asked him why he did not ask me first before entering my property. With his attitude and my attitude, it soon became a shoving and pushing angry scene. I dared him to hit me in the face. "Hit me, and see what fucking happens." I was in the **'survive and fight'** mode drilled into us by the Army. Deb came out and pulled me away and fortunately for me the young chippie left the scene. Later his boss came and apologised to me. But that was not the end of my **angry** outbursts. When the builders started hammering at six in the morning, I fronted the council and complained. For a short time after my complaint they started work at 7am which is the correct time but before long they were back at it again at 6am starts with sounds of electric saws and hammers banging. After a bad night with a **nightmare**, my **emotions** erupted. I got my axe, stormed outside and chopped all their wooden pegs inside my boundary and threw them back on their side. I yelled, "If you don't have any consideration, neither do I." That got the message across as I never heard a sound again after the incident.

> ***TV also has a powerful impact on my ability to manage my anger symptoms. I feel my mood swings dramatically when I watch news on politics and world events. I become seriously angry and depressed at the attitudes of different politicians and our involvement in wars overseas which leads to negative feelings including criticising people. Military training and war-time experiences have had a powerful effect on my beliefs about the world, my morals and values.***

For the rest of 2005 I was still struggling with **depression** and could not find the **motivation** to do anything. However, I gradually built up my strength and motivation from therapy treatment, counselling, family and friends. My Vietnam veteran mate, Nick Quigley, came to visit me and suggested I should **set goals for myself** like writing about my adventures down south and stop being so self-critical and give credit for what I have achieved. My family and friends all told me the same, they were envious of my experiences and opportunities to visit and live in Antarctica. Thanks to all the encouragement, I started thinking about my **negative** attitude and realised I had achieved everything I had set out to do. All this **positive** talk and thoughts inspired me to put pen to paper and write about my adventures down on the ice.

On the home front, Deb continued to work as a casual Teacher-Aide at the local Primary school, Michelle finally finished her degree and got a teaching job at Nanango High School (190 kilometres north-west of Brisbane) and David completed his third year at university in Civil Engineering.

With continuous physiotherapy for my head and neck injuries, at the beginning of 2006 I started to feel a lot better within myself with less headaches and more movement in my neck area. Even my PTSD symptoms had lessened off with weekly therapy treatment and counselling. Part of Dr Flanagan's therapy treatment was hypnosis to suppress my memories of Vietnam and modify my behaviour.

I would be exhausted after attending the weekly hypnosis program, so Deb would have to drive me home from Rockhampton.

With my health improved, I decided to get out of my comfort zone for the first time since I arrived home from Casey and take a four-wheel-drive road trip to Giles Weather Station which was celebrating its 50th Anniversary (2nd August) with Deb, David and a couple of mates. It was a wonderful two-week trip especially on the dirt tracks of the Plenty Highway (498 kilometres mostly unsealed road, from the Northern Territory/Queensland border to the Stuart Highway – 68 kilometres north of Alice Springs) and on the aborigine land between Alice Springs to Docker River to Giles. The only mishap on the trip was a punctured tyre at Jervois on the Plenty Highway. The reunion at the Weather Station went well and it gave me a different perspective about what it was like visiting the Station as a tourist. On the return trip we walked around the base of Ayers Rock which took around two hours and in Alice Springs I visited my father's grave and my old Primary school which I attended back in the fifties.

> ***Going on the trip re-energised me and uplifted my mood and feelings. It distracted my mind from my PTSD symptoms especially with my anxiety avoidance. The holiday was the first I spent with Debbie and David for more than two years while Michelle could not join us as she was working at Nanango High School. It was a special occasion.***

In October 2006, I attended my first 104 Sig Sqn reunion on the Gold Coast with Debbie and David for three days. It felt like I was in a time machine as I remembered those who served with me in Vietnam with young faces and now some thirty-six years on, with old faces. We chatted about the good times and the bad times in Vietnam and life since leaving the Army. On the last day, the RSL (Returned and Services League) unveiled a dedication plaque to all the Signal Units that served in Vietnam from 1965 to 1972 on the beach front park at Tweed Heads.

On Anzac Day 2007 I decided to march. This was the first time I got involved on Anzac Day since at Davis in 2003 where my fellow expeditioners respected me for serving my country and for the first time, I felt special and wanted. However, all this disappeared when a bloke questioned whether I was a true Vietnam veteran. As a veteran I wore my medals over my heart on the left side of my chest while relatives wore them on the right side. This bloke was wearing medals on his right chest and marching for a relative who had served during the Second World War. He asked me if I was marching for my dad. I replied, "No, for myself." He scoffed at me and raved on, "You mean your dad? You're too young to be a Vietnam veteran and you should be wearing those medals on the right side of your chest." A woman nearby piped up and agreed with him. "No, I am a Vietnam veteran," I pleaded. I felt embarrassed and fumbled for my wallet to prove my veteran status with my DVA Gold Card as the march began.

> ***I promised myself I would never march again after that humiliation. I have heard similar stories from our women veterans.***

My **anxiety** could be brought on by so many unexpected elements that I found it difficult to manage those events. In winter 2007, I came down with a bad dose of the flu, with a sore throat and blocked nose. I could not breathe properly, and I had the same feeling when my pit hole collapsed on top of me and almost suffocated me in Vietnam. For five days I could not sleep. I tried reading, listened to music, watched TV, but every time I was about to go to sleep, I had flashbacks or anxiety attacks. Dr Flanagan wanted to hospitalise me to induce sleep. He believed the flu had possibly triggered too many chemicals in my brain. I refused to go into hospital, so the other alternative was a heavy dose of sleeping tablets.

> ***Fortunately, the tablets worked, and I recovered before I nearly lost the plot altogether.***

In late 2007 I contacted Scotty Wilson's family through DVA. I always felt guilty for not contacting his mum and dad after his death in Vietnam 1971, particularly as Scotty was my best mate. On the 2nd March 2008, I finally met his two sisters, Helen and Morag, but sadly Scotty's parents had passed away. It was an emotional reunion, particularly when I presented each sister with a collection of coloured and black and white photos in a large frame. In the frame there were nine photos of Scotty, a rising sun badge, his medal ribbons and two poppies, all on a green background and encased in a dark brown wooden frame.

> ***On every Anzac Day I contact Helen and Morag and wish them all the best and tell them my thoughts are always with them and their brother, Scotty.***

Over the years, I feel I had become emotionally detached and increasingly distrustful of other people. I was badly hurt by the public reaction during and after the Vietnam War, and I became

protective of myself and family. My closest friends are all veteran mates with whom I served in Vietnam.

The Vietnam War established life-long feelings of intense loyalty, trust and mateship. It was a defining moment in our lives as young men as we experienced the persistent threat of attack and the risk of being killed or wounded. After the war, we all had to cope with a feeling of profound disillusionment and having experienced the dangers of war, life was an anti-climax. We also suffered from the ugly and traitorous behaviour of the Australian public towards us and the Vietnam War. These feelings brought us even closer and bonded us for life.

In March 2008 I travelled to Ballina from Yeppoon to visit my dying Nui Dat tent mate Wayne Hackett. Wayne had mouth and throat cancer, and I visited him in his caravan at a local park. It was an emotional final meeting. He was skin and bone and could not talk.

When I left, I embraced Wayne for the last time. We both cried as his weak, skeletal body embraced mine in a final farewell hug.

> ***Wayne died a few weeks later, after having discharged himself from hospital. He took a taxi to the caravan park, had a shower, got into brand new pyjamas and died peacefully in his own bed.***

The day before Anzac Day 2008, I had been invited to my old High School in Caloundra to lay a wreath at their Anzac Day ceremony. Apparently, I was the only student to serve in the Vietnam War. When I attended the school in the sixties there were only about 80 students, now there are more than a thousand.

On my way to the school I had a panic attack. For twenty minutes I sat in my vehicle on the side of the road as panic engulfed me in waves, each more forceful than the last.

> ***Panic attacks are episodes of severe anxiety which can occur quite suddenly. They are extremely distressing and last for just a few minutes or much longer. At the time, my symptoms were: light-headedness, shaking, dry mouth, difficulty in gathering my thoughts, pounding heart, sweating and an urge to flee.***

Somehow, I made it to the main gate of the school where the Principal and a school Prefect welcomed me. During the ceremony I donated two books to their library. After the ceremony I adjourned to the staff room for a cuppa and chat with teachers and students and afterwards toured the school. This was the second time I felt appreciated since I returned home from Vietnam in 1970. The first time was in Antarctica in 2003.

I was honoured to be back at my old school, delighted to have the opportunity to stand tall before all those young faces. Feeling exhausted, I realised for the umpteenth time what a toll Vietnam had taken of me and my family. I had taken another step on a journey that had barely begun.

> ***Every year since 2008, I have attended the Caloundra High School Anzac Day ceremony and presented the school with two Military History books for their library.***

In June 2008 Deb, David and I flew to England for a six-week family holiday. Michelle couldn't join us as she was teaching at Baralaba State School in Central Queensland. When flying

I usually take **anxiety tablets** to calm myself down. I took two **ALEPAM-15MG tablets** which caused me drowsiness. The closed confined space of the aircraft did not help me with my **anxiety**, especially when the sound of the cabin door closed reminding me of feeling trapped in the aircraft like I was in my pit hole. On the Singapore to London leg of the flight, I had a severe nightmare screaming out which disturbed nearby passengers. Luckily, I was sitting between Deb and David and they calmed me down.

While in London I had a panic attack on a tube train when a large crowd of passengers boarded. I felt trapped and had trouble breathing, a feeling of being choked. Deb and David noticed my condition and managed to get me off the train.

Over the next weeks, we hired a car. I drove while David navigated with Deb in the back seat. We toured Plymouth, the Cornish coast, then up into Wales and visited plenty of castles. Back into England to Chester where I visited my Great-Grandfather's grave. We took a fast ferry to Ireland, where again we hired a car in Dublin and toured the southwest coastal towns, the Ring of Kerry, Killarney National Park, Cliffs of Moher, Tipperary where my Great-Grandmother was born and finally back to Dublin. Then we went back to Holyhead in Wales by ferry and hired another car, to Manchester, North Sea coast, Yorkshire Dales, Lake country, Hadrian's Wall, onto Scotland-Loch Ness, and finally back to Carlisle, England where we caught a train to London then onto Paris on the Eurostar for a couple of days. We flew back to Australia from Heathrow Airport via Singapore on the 24th July.

It was an enjoyable holiday, but the most frustrating part was driving on the narrow country roads through villages and small towns, especially the busy round-abouts. I was glad David was with me because I believe I would not have made it with my anxiety. Being tired from driving and sleeping in unfamiliar beds caused a lot of nightmares for me on the trip.

In August after getting over our UK trip, David and I were on the road again to Canberra and on the 18th attended the Vietnam Veterans Remembrance Day service held at the Vietnam Memorial in Anzac parade where the Prime Minister Rudd attended. The next day we attended the unveiling of a plaque for our Signal units in Vietnam in the western courtyard at the Australian War Memorial (AWM). It was full on catching up with old mates that I had served with in Vietnam. On our final day we toured the AWM and we placed a red poppy next to Scotty Wilson's name, my best mate killed in Vietnam, and Eddie Clifton's name. Eddy was the son of my father's older sister, Muriel. Born in Adelaide on 1 July 1922, he enlisted in the AIF in 1940 with a mate and both lied about their ages. Eddy sailed from Australia on 28 December 1940 and celebrated his nineteenth birthday overseas. Killed in action at Tobruk on 3 August 1941, my first cousin is buried at Tobruk War Cemetery. I have a photo of him in his Army uniform, and on every Anzac Day I lay a wreath in memory of him and Scotty Wilson.

On the 23rd September, we attended David's graduation ceremony in Rockhampton. David graduated with first class honours as a Bachelor of Civil Engineering. At the end of the school year, Michelle quit her teaching job at Baralaba

State School because of issues with accommodation and kid's behaviour.

At the beginning of 2009, we all decided to move into our new house in Palmwoods on the Sunshine Coast which we had purchased in February 2008. With the downturn of the housing market we decided to keep the Yeppoon house and rent it out.

David got a job with Leighton's Engineering in the city but only lasted in that job for six weeks before joining Queensland Rail as a Graduate Civil Engineer, while Michelle got teaching contract work on the coast and wanted to study part time Environment Health at university. In July David shifted into his own house at Narangba located 34 km north of Brisbane which he purchased through the First Home Buyer's grant.

After settling into our new surrounds, in November I went into Nambour Selangor Hospital for a hernia operation, my second, but this one was by keyhole through my belly button. While in hospital, I had one of my worst nightmares. After the operation they put me into a four-bed male ward with a hernia operation patient next to me and two knee replacement patients opposite. Both these patients were connected to foot-pump machines, which emitted a noise every few minutes. At around 11.00pm a nurse came into the ward and pulled a pale green curtain around my bed and turned the lights off. There was still dull light shining into the ward from the hallway. I must have fallen asleep as I later found myself screaming and shaking in terror on the ward floor.

My intensely vivid nightmare: I was surrounded by the jungle foliage in Vietnam which was the pale green curtain and the pump machines sounded like noises coming from the jungle.

The other patients in the ward must have wondered what was going on as the nurses escorted me away to a single ward.

On the 5th January 2010 I visited my dying Vietnam mate Tom Spark in Ipswich hospital. He had lived in the same tent with me when we were at Nui Dat. It was an emotional last farewell as Tom gripped my right hand for at least twenty minutes before his grip slowly weakened as he went into a permanent deep sleep. Tom passed away on the 12th January, only 61 years of age. I attended his funeral on the 15th January and met up with other Vietnam mates whom I served with.

Tom was my third tent mate at Nui Dat to pass away, following Russell Pye from a heart attack and Wayne Hackett from cancer. The other tent mates alive are Boobla Hegarty, Terry Skinner and Nev Roberts.

Tom died from aggressive bowel cancer. He was only five days younger than me. To this day I wonder if the Agent Orange-herbicide they were spraying or the anti-malaria tablets of Paludrine and Dapsone we were taking whilst in Vietnam had caused his cancer. There are reports that the cancer rate of Vietnam veterans is significantly higher than in the Australian population.

After four years of putting pen to paper, in late August 2010 my book *Ice Journey* was published by Big Sky Publishing. I had to do a couple of talks with the media and visit libraries promoting my book and talk about my ongoing battle with PTSD.

David went on holidays to America and Canada from the 28th April to the 4th June to get away from bullying in his toxic workplace. After he returned to the workshop, the bullying continued so David walked out from his job on the 13th August, his birthday and refused to return to work until Queensland Rail found him another position away from the workshop.

Deb and I had arranged a house swap holiday with our home in Palmwoods to an apartment on the River Thames in the heart of London. We suggested David to join us to get away from his current ugly situation. On the 6th September we flew from Brisbane via Singapore to London. The house swap period was for three weeks so most of the time Deb and I stayed in London while David went to Switzerland for a week. When he got back, we hired a car for three days and toured the sea resort towns of Brighton and Dover. When the time period expired in the apartment, Deb and I travelled by train to Switzerland and visited Geneva and Montreux, a Swiss town on the shoreline of Lake Geneva at the foot of the Alps while David toured Scotland. After visiting our different holiday areas, we all flew back home on the 4th October.

David started back at work on the 28th October in the Design Office, Queensland Rail in the city. He was now living at home with us at Palmwoods and would commute to the city and back to Palmwoods station by train during the week. For a short period, David was ok then became depressed and angry again. For the first time I realised my PTSD had impacted my family. As a father I had become over-protective with my children and when they went out into the big wide world they struggled. The whole family had to put up with my nightmares, depression, anger outbursts, mood swings and nit-picking for years. I would pick on small issues like dirty marks on fridge doors, crumbs on the table, chairs left out of the table, strict eating diets and strict time schedules like on our road trips and from social outings. I had brought them up in a world of military discipline of drill, drill and drill in study and education.

I never thought about their feelings, only my own. It was all about me. The Army had trained me well, either to kill or obey orders but they forgot to de-train me when I went back to civilian life and that is where the problem started. David was diagnosed and treated for a derivative form of PTSD. I wanted David to get help and counselling, so I contacted the Vietnam Veterans Counselling Service (VVCS) in Maroochydore and Deb, David and I fronted the Counselling service on the 10th November for the first time. David continued with a couple more sessions for the next month.

David quit his job with QR – Queensland Rail and left Australia on the 23rd February 2011 on a flight to the United States, a one-way ticket to Helena, Montana.

I was heartbroken as I watched my little boy, now a young man as he disappeared down the Brisbane Airport terminal corridor to board his flight. He was following my journey thirty-six years earlier when I left Australia emotionally broken from war and burdened with PTSD looking for a new way of life. He was doing the same, emotionally broken from bullying in the workplace and burdened with a derivative form of PTSD caused by me. It was a sad emotional day for all of us. I cried all the way home to Palmwoods. It was the same feeling when my mum passed away.

The stress impact of war affects the majority of veterans' children. It is like throwing a rock into a water pool and it ripples out.

I entered another black hole after David's departure and as I had left Yeppoon, I had to find another Psychiatrist. I found Dr Paul Cadzow from the yellow pages and soon I was having weekly counselling sessions. He put me on different medication from my previous Psychiatrist. I was now on Escitalopram 20mg and Seroquel 100mg for sleeping.

Dr Cadzow encouraged me to set small goals for myself to get out of my depression. In March I decided to drive down to Victoria for two weeks and visit friends and a cousin. I visited my Vietnam mates that I had not seen since Vietnam, Richard Burgess at Koonoomoo over the Victorian border from New South Wales, Leigh Bennett in Echuca and Bluey Baird in Mildura. I also visited my cousin Robyn in Daylesford and caught up with Gerbil, the Antarctica cook who I was with at Macquarie Island and Davis. The trip improved my mental well-being. I continued to occupy myself on my return home by visiting twelve libraries over the next few months on the Sunshine Coast and the Moreton Bay Region promoting my book *Ice Journey*.

David arrived in Helena, Montana when Ron and Sandy were still on holidays, so he stayed with other friends, Tucker and Annie until they arrived home. While at Tucker's place he purchased a 1984 Cadillac Coupe Deville for around 2500 US dollars. The Caddy was in good condition and only required four new tyres and some mechanical work, which Tucker carried out. Just as they had helped me, Ron and Sandy and friends looked after David and took him horse riding, cross country skiing and other activities. After staying a month with Ron and Sandy, David was offered a job on 2nd April in Calgary, Alberta, Canada working as a Rail Engineer. His job was to work and supervise at different sites, building new and upgrading rail lines with the Canadian Pacific Railway within and outside the Calgary area. He soon shifted into a share house with another young guy and had his own toilet and bathroom.

David wanted us to visit him in Calgary, so we decided to fly to Calgary on the 12th August. Unfortunately, Michelle could not join us as she was still studying part time at university for an Environmental Health degree. Deb and I arrived in Calgary on David's birthday the 13th.

David arrived in his caddy to pick us up at the airport. It had been six months since we last saw him, then depressed and aggressive, now an assertive confident young man. Like me he had turned his life around with support from Ron and Sandy and friends, but the biggest positive was respect from his co-workers within his workplace. We were in Calgary for eleven weeks and rented an apartment about 30 minutes walking distance from downtown Calgary. Most days we would walk along the Bow River to downtown, view the shops, have a bite to eat, relax somewhere along the river or in parks and return to the apartment.

> *It was good exercise with over an hour's walk. I found exercise improved PTSD symptoms like my moods, decreased my anxiety and improved my sleep. It was the first time since I left work I was doing regular exercise and I felt good.*

We would catch up with David on most days during the week for lunch or dinner. For the weekends he would take us either to his place or a friend's place for a barbeque. He also drove us to different Calgary tourist spots and on one trip he drove us to the Banff National Park where we visited the spectacular Bow River Falls and Lake Moraine. Whilst in Calgary we managed to visit Ron and Sandy for a week when we hired a car. It was a great holiday but as they say, 'All Good Things Must Come to An End'. After an emotion farewell with David, we departed Calgary on the 25th October for home.

It was not long after, on December the 1st, David was transferred with the Engineering Firm to London to take up a similar position as a Structural Engineer designing and inspecting different structures within London and the UK. He was now trying to get familiar with London.

Michelle, after not coping with school teaching, completed her Environmental Health Degree with Honours at the end of 2011 term and continued with part time work for EnviroCom on the Sunshine Coast, teaching schools on environmental topics.

On the 12th March 2012, Deb and I attended for the first time a VVCS-Lifestyle Workshop at a Noosa resort for five days to help veterans to live a better lifestyle by understanding what PTSD is, diet and nutrition, ways to have a better relationship, relaxation methods, and finding solutions and setting goals. We found it was beneficial to us and for the first time realised there were people just like us struggling with PTSD in their relationship and in the family.

Unfortunately, I had a nightmare every night while at the resort, stirred by stories from other veterans and partners attending the Lifestyle Workshop.

I found I was dealing with my PTSD symptoms much better probably due to visiting libraries and Probus and Lions clubs, talking about my issues and symptoms. All up I did fourteen talks in 2012 from the South Burnett Region to the Gold Coast in Queensland and to the North Coast towns of New South Wales.

On the 24th September Michelle started her new job as an Environmental/Health officer with the Moreton Bay Shire Council at Caboolture. Her new job was to inspect new food businesses and see if they are aligned with state health regulations laws.

Another highlight for us during 2012, was when David completed the Dublin marathon on the 28th October in under 5 hours (4 hrs 58 mins 40 secs). He texted me, *'I survived. It was the hardest physical challenge I have ever done. I am extremely sore.'*

David returned home on the 5th December for the Christmas and New Year break and to renew his working visa for UK. It was good to have the whole family home for Christmas and New Year, but the New Year's Eve celebrations did not go well for me.

We all headed to Mooloolaba beach to see the New Year in with fireworks on display. I thought I could handle the loud cracking and bright flashing of the fireworks, but as soon as the fireworks started, I had a complete meltdown of anxiety attacks and flashbacks. I was reliving Vietnam again. I had no control with my body shaking violently. The family escorted me away from the beach and headed home.

I should have taken notice of my previous experiences when watching the fireworks on TV. I always had panic attacks and had to leave.

In early 2013 we decided to sell the Palmwoods house. We discovered there was a major problem with leaves and branches falling into my property from the forest reserve next door and the neighbour's property at the back. I was continuously cleaning leaves from the roof and gutters of the house, the swimming pool, lawns and pathways and this triggered my PTSD symptoms of becoming irritable, frustrated and angry. It all started when I came home and found my pool full of leaves from my back-door neighbour's trees. Prior, I had been asking him for some time to trim his trees, but he always ignored my requests. I fronted him at his front door and asked him to look at my pool, but he refused. He told me to get off of his property and pushed me and this triggered my anger. I vigorously pushed him back through the entry of his front door and then he threatened to call the police, but he never did. At about the same time I was in arguments with the council, asking them to remove some of the big gum trees near my side fence but once again my pleas fell on deaf ears. The final straw came on January the 26th and 27th when ex-cyclone Oswald hit the Sunshine Coast with destructive winds and torrential rain and caused a lot of damage with large trees blown over including branches into my property from the forest reserve. There were branches everywhere, on my roof, in my swimming pool and yard and to top it all off, we had no power for three days. Fortunately, David was home, and he helped me to clean up the mess. It took us two days to clean up the debris of broken branches.

With all the stress and uncertainty of the house, I frequently found I was having dizzy spells, headaches and difficulty in digesting my food, as well having more nightmares. Once again, I had to go and see Dr Cadzow for help.

CHAPTER 27

With great relief we sold the house on the 22nd March about nine thousand dollars below our asking price.

After gaining his UK working visa David departed Brisbane on the 9th April for London, and it was again another emotional farewell. It was all happening when on the next day Deb and I signed a contract for a four-bedroom house with swimming pool at Pelican Waters. This time we made sure there were no gum trees nearby.

We moved out of the Palmwoods house on the 29th April and had to put our furniture and belongings into a storage until we could move into our new house. In the meantime, we moved into a holiday unit at Kings Beach Caloundra.

On the 20th May we finally moved into our new home. Just as well because I was struggling with the confined spaces of the holiday unit causing increase nightmares and lack of sleep.

I felt claustrophobic all the time in the unit.

Although the house was only five years old, we upgraded it to our liking with new carpet, blinds, solar hot water, cemented the inside shed area and closed the back area with large sliding doors.

In October 2013, I was asked to visit libraries in Victoria to talk about my PTSD for mental health week. We visited nine towns along the Goulburn River and the Murray River in northern Victoria including my old hometown of Echuca.

At the libraries, I met many people like me suffering from mental health problems with amazing sad stories.

The year went quickly. In late November Michelle and her partner Neil moved into their new house at North Lakes and on the 8th December David arrived home for his Christmas and New Year holiday break. We were kept busy and active for the month while he was home. We went surfing at Kings beach Caloundra, we climbed Mt Coolum (208m or 682.4 feet) and went on a seven-day road trip along the scenic New South Wales coast all the way down to Eden on the South Coast and then returned home. David flew back to London on the 12th January 2014 to his job.

I had contacted and met up with my local federal member Alex Somlyay a few months back regarding my sexual assault while in the Army. I wanted to know how to report the incident to the Defence Abuse Response Taskforce (DART). Soon after Mr Somlyay sent me a report form to be filled out on the sexual assault incident and signed by a Justice of Peace (JP) and forwarded to DART. I did all this in 2013.

DART was established on 26th November 2012 to assist complainants who had suffered sexual abuse, physical abuse, sexual harassment and workplace harassment and bullying in Defence prior to the 11th April 2011. I first heard about the Taskforce when watching television, where a young woman victim spoke publicly for the first time about her ordeal in the now infamous Australian Defence Force Academy (ADFA) Skype sex scandal on the ABC's 7.30 Report in November 2013.

After forty-five years I wanted justice. I felt my sexual assault by this sick sex predator back in 1968 had caused negative feelings within myself over the years, such as anger, disgust and guilt. I always felt dirty when having sex,

my mind emotionally distant or not present during sex and sometimes I avoided it altogether. It was one of the reasons why I left the Army because I became too sensitive and I wanted to distance myself not only from the memory but also the uniform that the predator represented.

Soon afterwards I was contacted by a DART Case Coordinator to discuss my case and he passed back to the Taskforce the information I gave him about my sexual assault. I received a letter from DART on the 24th February 2014 acknowledging my abuse case and providing information about the outcomes available to me. I was offered:

- referral to counselling services;
- a Reparation Payment of $50,000;
- referral of appropriate matters to police or military justice authorities for formal criminal investigation and assessment for prosecution;
- participation in a restorative engagement process with an appropriate senior Defence member to acknowledge harm caused.

On the 28th November 2014, I met up with my DART facilitator, Callum Campbell, to talk about restorative process with my health and well-being for the future. A few months earlier, I had attended the Caloundra Police Station where I provided a written statement about the assault. On the 8th December two detectives from the Frankston Criminal Investigation Branch (CIB) in Victoria visited me at home to investigate my statement. I had to view and identify the suspected predator from photos taken years earlier. In the end, I failed to give a positive identification. The case is still open at Frankston CIB. Although I was disappointed with the identification as I thought it would have been easier, the whole DART process came to an end the next day on the 9th December when I met up with Callum Campbell and Brigadier Stephen Beaumont at Rydges resort in Caloundra. The Brigadier, in his uniform, apologised to me for the sexual abuse I suffered at the School of Signals in 1968 and said the Army was determined to change the present Army culture to a respectful cohesive culture, where abuse of any sort plays no part. He said hearing my story reinforces the importance of the culture change and promised me that I would receive an apology from the Chief of Army soon. The letter arrived in late February 2015. From the typed letter :-

> *In my capacity as Chief of Army, I apologise to you unreservedly for the sexual assault that was perpetrated against you while you were undergoing training at the School of Signals, Balcombe. I offer this apology in the hope it assists in healing the emotional scars that you have carried for so long. I trust you can appreciate my commitment as Chief of Army to assist those Army members who have suffered abuse in the past, and my commitment to eliminate the conditions that might lead to the existence and tolerance of such behaviour today and into the future.*

In his own writing at the end of letter :-

> *My heartfelt apologies again and with deep respect.*
>
> *Signed : D.L. Morrison, AO, Lieutenant General, Chief of Army. 23rd February 2015.*

On 25 January 2016, Morrison was made Australian of the Year. At least I received some justice, more than other victims. I still get angry especially when I am watching television news on sexual abuse cases in Australia and around the world.

In 2013, the Gallipoli Medical Research Foundation (GMRF) and the Returned and Services League (RSL) commenced a project called 'PTSD Initiative' to help veterans and their families. The research project was to investigate the physical and psychological toll of PTSD in Vietnam veterans. They were looking for 300 Vietnam veterans in total to participate, 150 with and 150 without PTSD, for the study. I volunteered to be one of the participants with PTSD. After signing a consent form, on the 28th April 2014, I drove to the GMRF at Greenslopes hospital for an interview on my medical history plus breathing and kidney tests for the research program. Over the following weeks I went back three times to the GMRF for further tests and interviews. The study was to continue for at least another year before the final report was completed.

In July 2014 Dr Cadzow was not happy with my lack of sleep so he referred me to a Sleep Specialist in Caloundra. On August 20th I went into Buderim hospital for an overnight sleep study. The nurse attached wires all over my head and body. This triggered anxiety attacks all through the night. I could not sleep with those wires hanging off me. The nurse kept coming into the room saying, "get to sleep". When I fronted the Sleep Specialist a week later, he was quite abrupt with me. "What a waste time. I have insufficient data as you did not sleep. I can't help you. Go back to your Psych doctor." His attitude, thinking it was my fault, pissed me off. Obviously, he did not understand the symptoms of PTSD.

My second book, *My Vietnam War_Scarred Forever,* was published and launched in early September 2014, so over the coming weeks I did newspaper and media interviews. I decided to donate a percentage of my royalties to Soldier On an organisation that helps our young war veterans.

David and his partner Louise arrived home on the 8th February 2015. He had quit his job in London and wanted to work either in Australia or New Zealand. David met Louise, who is a school music teacher, in July 2013. They both departed for Wellington, New Zealand in May when David was offered work for a Civil Engineering Firm.

David was coping well with his derivative PTSD. I was relieved that he was closer to home.

2015 was a busy year for us. With my second book published, Deb and I drove down to Victoria and South Australia for seventeen days in April to promote it. We visited eight different libraries and did three media talks on our tour to both States, but no doubt the highlight for us was visiting the eye-catching Seymour Vietnam Veterans Commemorative Walk where I viewed the honour wall detailing the names of those who fell during the conflict and the many other walls detailing the names of all who served in the Vietnam war including my name with excellent images on the background of each wall. Other highlights were visiting the National Vietnam Veterans Museum at Phillip Island, and the stunning scenery and lookouts along the Great Ocean Road which was built by returned soldiers between 1919 and 1932 and dedicated to soldiers killed during World War 1. Another special memory was spending ANZAC day with mates in my old hometown of Echuca. On my tour, I met a lot of people with PTSD including a former policewoman who was involved in the Russell Street bombing in March 1986 where a policewoman was killed, and 22 people injured.

> ***The negative for me was those stories brought on more nightmares. I had 8 while on the tour.***

CHAPTER 28

PTSD PROGRAMMES AND CHALLENGES

Dr Cadzow was worried about my lack of sleep and nightmares, so he wanted me to attend a PTSD Programme at Greenslopes Private Hospital for two days per week, Wednesday and Thursday, beginning 15th July. Along with six other veterans including three young veterans from the Afghanistan war, I attended the programme for ten weeks. We had daily counselling and sessions on relaxation, alcohol management, relationship skills, living skills, sleep management, exercise and psychology – comprising cognitive behaviour therapy, depression, anxiety and anger.

At the end of course I felt I had benefited, especially learning new strategies to put in place like Mindfulness and Cognitive behaviour therapy (CBT).

On the 10th November, Deb and I flew to New Zealand for two weeks to visit David and Louise and to tour parts of the South Island. I had visited New Zealand back in 1973 with my twin brother Don and mate Stephen Smyth but it was the first time for Deb. For our seven day trip to the South Island we boarded a ferry from Wellington across Cook Strait to Picton and there we hired a car and drove to Westport on the west coast, to Punakaiki – viewed Pancake Rocks – to Greymouth, across Arthur's Pass in the Southern Alps, to Kaikoura on the east coast, to Nelson on Tasman Bay, finally back to Picton and onto the ferry back to Wellington.

It was a great two-week holiday especially spending time with David and Louise.

My dear sister Patsy, eight years older than me passed away on the 12th April 2016 from emphysema. She donated her body to Medical Science. I last spoke to Patsy on the 8th and she knew she did not have long to live. All her family including my twin brother were at her bedside when she passed away. I did not go to Perth to see her because it was her wish for me to not see her in her present frail condition as I was close to her. Patsy lived a sad life, she was abused and bashed by two husbands which impacted her life and plummeted her family into tough hard times. She loved her family and in her last few years found great happiness when she was with her little granddaughter, Danielle.

On my many talks at libraries I met a lot of women with PTSD from domestic violence.

For 2016 Anzac Day service I got involved for the first time with the day service by driving, in my 1967 Cadillac Coupe Deville, a couple of disabled old veterans who could not march. David and I purchased the Caddy in October 2008 from a Classic car dealer on the Gold Coast who shipped it in from the United States.

I have never marched, only attended Dawn Services, since the Anzac Day service at Yeppoon when I was humiliated and embarrassed by a non-veteran who accused me of not being a true veteran and for wearing my medals on the incorrect side of my chest. After almost four decades, I noticed for the first time after attending the 2016 Anzac Day Service march, the public perception has changed towards us Vietnam veterans particularly with the growing number of people attending Anzac Day marches.

> ***Since 2016 I have driven disabled veterans in my Cadillac on every Anzac Day.***

The PTSD Programme at Greenslopes Private Hospital introduced me to Mates4Mates and shortly afterwards I signed up. The organisation helps the lives of current and ex-serving Australian Defence Force members and their families impacted by service. They provide physical, psychological and social support services to improve the wellbeing of all members.

Deb and I attended a Mates4Mates Equine Therapy Couple's program in May for five days set in the Gold Coast hinterland. Our accommodation was at Bartle House near Tamborine Mountain and the horse ranch was near Canungra. The program was to help couples with their relationship and learn new strategies of coping with PTSD. Apparently, horses can mirror the people they are with, read people minds and help with physical and emotional needs. They can sense our feelings, read our body language with our heartbeats, our facial expressions, our breathing and are sensitive to the surrounding environment.

When we arrived at the horse yards, I was a bit apprehensive at first and did not know what to expect. Amazingly, Gemma, a mare, walked up to me while Mr Hobbs, a gelding, bonded with Deb. Over the four days at the horse ranch we slowly built a close, trusting relationship with our horses. Activities included learning basic horsemanship like handling and leading the horses. We learnt how to brush and groom, how to put a bridle on a horse, how to lead the horse by walking forward and backwards, how to walk and jog with the horse, with and without rope, how to turn the horse in a circle with rope over low lying logs and how to feed a horse. At Bartle House we had counselling sessions in the evening, learning to recognise our negative thought patterns and behaviour and to develop new positive thoughts with help from Mates4Mates psychologists and from our experiences interacting with the horses. We also did a lot of other activities like working on love languages and practising mindfulness.

After attending the Equine Therapy program Deb and I felt we learnt a lot from the program about how to calm ourselves in stressful situations and improve our communication and trust in our relationship. It was an amazing experience and gave me a different perspective towards horses, especially how intelligent and strong they are. Gemma was a former racehorse while Mr Hobbs was a

pet horse on a farm and was abused by his male owner with whip scars obvious on his face area. We were told Mr Hobbs never bonded with male participants on the Equine Therapy program.

Not long after that program, I applied to walk the Kokoda Track with Mates4Mates rehabilitation challenge, and I was successful. My main motivation was to confront my fears and to get out of my comfort zone and walk for my best mate Robert 'Scotty' Wilson who was killed in Vietnam, my other Vietnam mates who have died since, and to honour our soldiers who fought to save our country. Leading up to the walk, I did 17 weeks of training, walking up and down hills on the coastal strip of Caloundra, clocking up 1,141kms in 238 hours. I also spent 21 hours in the gym, strengthening my body with my exercise physiologist at Resolve Fitness. The Kokoda adventure started on Thursday the 13th October at the Mates4Mates building where I met up with twelve fellow trekkers and two team leaders at a pre-departure briefing and welcome barbecue. The next morning, we flew from Brisbane to Port Moresby, arriving in the early afternoon, then proceeded to our accommodation at Crowne Plaza where we were briefed and issued with our gear.

Day one:

Started early when we flew from Port Moresby to Popondetta arriving at 7am. From there we travelled by trucks on rough dirt roads to Kokoda (340m above sea level). Before we set off at midday, we visited the Kokoda memorial. We climbed steadily for three hours in hot and humid conditions, along the, at times, steep track with most of us finding it difficult. My porter,

Billy, was constantly pouring cold water over my head to cool me off. We reached our overnight destination, a small village called Deniki (895m) where we found our tents already set up by our porters. We washed under the village water pipe. There were thunderstorms all night, so I did not sleep well. Going to the toilet was a hazardous exercise as you had to navigate on a slippery narrow track with steep drop-offs. The toilets were all similar on the track, in small outhouses with a dunny seat over a large pit-hole. For our meals we had ration packs with a variety of food which was issued daily. For our evening meals we would put our rice/pasta packets together and the porters heated it in a large pot. Any food left over from my ration pack I would give to my porter, Billy.

Day two:
We were up early at 4am to get on the track at 6am. For the first hour the walk was extremely hard with steep climbs but after a while it became undulating with up and down hills. At lunch we visited the Isurava memorial battlefield site where our Trek leader, Glenn, gave us a rundown on the history of the battle. Isurava was the site of some of the most intense fighting in the Kokoda Track campaign. The memorial features four Australian black granite pillars that are each inscribed with a single word: **'Courage', 'Endurance', 'Mateship', and 'Sacrifice'** representing the values and qualities of those Australian soldiers who fought along the Kokoda Track. In the afternoon I nearly fell into a creek, but Billy saved me. After nine hours on the track we arrived late afternoon at Alola (1340m). I did not feel so exhausted probably because it was

overcast, and we trekked mainly under the jungle canopy. Again, it rained during the night.

Day three:

On the track by 6am. It was an extremely hard walk on the slippery muddy track. I had to concentrate with every step I took as there were big drops off the narrow track. After a couple of gruelling hours, one of our trekkers, a veteran, collapsed, suffering from body fatigue and heat exhaustion. He could not go any further, so it was decided to medevac him out by helicopter to Port Moresby, accompanied by Trek leader, Alyssa. (Alyssa rejoined us in a couple days' time when the helicopter returned with our food supplies.) We continued and crossed the fast-flowing Eora Creek by a bridge made from branches and vines. I viewed a memorial plaque stating, **"The Eora Creek crossing represented one of the best defensive positions on the Kokoda Trail"** and nearby we viewed a Japanese ammunition cache of grenades and mortar shells. After more than ten hours on the track we made it to Templeton's Crossing No 2 (1700m). Late in the afternoon we all bathed in the creek which I found very refreshing and invigorating. Before dinner I joined others sitting down on a log and as soon as I sat down on the top end of the log it collapsed, causing me to fall down a steep slope. As I rolled down the slope my tail bone hit a broken stump, and this caused me extreme pain in the tail bone (Coccyx) for the following days on the track.

Day four:

We left Templeton's Crossing at 6am. For the first hour we trekked up a steep hill then, of course, went downhill, very steeply at times and slippery especially on the tree roots that spread out on the clay soil of the track. We had a lunch break at Naduri. After lunch we trekked further down a slippery steep track in a thunderstorm, followed by a gruelling high climb up to Launumu and, (surprise) a final steep downhill stretch to Efogi (1350m), arriving late afternoon. At Efogi, I viewed a sign indicating we were 48.1 kms from Kokoda and 45.5 kms to Owers Corner, so we had trekked more than halfway to our destination. In the evening it was my turn to talk about my life journey with PTSD and what I hoped to get out of walking the Kokoda Track.

Day five:

I woke feeling sick and lightheaded, so Glenn gave me some tablets for nausea. We started the trek early, up a steep hill then down a low decent for an emotional service at Mission Ridge. We continued to Brigade Hill where the Australian and Papua New Guinea flags were raised with a memorial plaque in between. On the memorial plaque I read **"This hill over which you walk was the site where one thousand Australians temporarily held back a much larger Japanese force advancing towards Port Moresby. In bitter fighting many men of both sides died. Today only their dust and the memories of their sacrifices remain"**. A service was held with poems, the Ode and the Australian and the Papua New Guinea (PNG) national anthems sung by us and our porters.

We then trekked to Menari for lunch followed by a tough trek up a steep hill where I struggled to reach the top and was relieved it was all downhill to Brown River (745m) for the night with a swim and wash in the river to freshen up.

Day six:

I was still feeling sick. We departed Brown River at 6am. It was a massive and challenging day for us all as we had to overcome the nine peaks or the false peaks. During the trek I counted nine peaks, but others said it was only five with four to go. The nine peaks seem to go on forever and my condition did not help as I was sick on the track a few times. We reached the peak and there was still debate about how many peaks we had climbed (too many!). In the mid-afternoon we crossed a creek in bare feet with our boots off. I found it very slippery on the rocks and at times Billy had to keep me upright and prevent me from slipping over into the creek. Our final challenge for the day was climbing Iribaiwa Ridge (900m) then downhill to Iribaiwa village. It was a long exhausting day, more than eleven hours on the track. The only food I could eat and keep down was bananas purchased from villages on the track. Every night on the track I would wash my clothes and Billy would dry them, including my boots, in front of the fire during the night.

Day seven:

I was still feeling sick and lightheaded, so bad I had to be helped to my feet. Glenn, the track leader gave me a couple of tablets to get me on my way and suggested I should give Billy my backpack for him to carry but I refused. We left Iribaiwa village at 6.30am and our main challenge was to climb the Golden Staircase. Glenn suggested we could do this individually at our own rate. It became a friendly race to the top with one of the young porters coming in first place while the first from our group made it in 29 minutes. I was one of the last to the top in 55 minutes. We trekked in wet boots all day as we crossed at least twenty creeks, some fast flowing and waist high. We arrived at Goldie River (420m) at 3.30pm and the early time gave us an opportunity to swim in the river. It was fast flowing and so refreshing I stayed in for at least 40 minutes. After the swim, my body and mind seemed to be reinvigorated, helped, I must admit, by the knowledge that we had only about another hour's walk to reach our destination the next day.

Day eight:

We woke this morning with our porters singing hymns. I took in the present moment with the beautiful blended sound and tone of their choir-like voices and the smell of the clear jungle air, along with the background sound of the river. My mind and heart felt the emotion as the images flowed within me – our Fuzzy Wuzzy Angels sang like their forefathers did when they assisted and escorted our injured troops along the Kokoda trail. Glenn took off early to put our flag and the PNG flag up on the track about 10 minutes from the top at Owers Corner (885m). We trekked up the final steep hill which took us about 45 minutes to reach the flags where we took photos including one of our Army teddy bear mascot called Franklin hanging on to the Australian flag. As we carried the flags up front, we reached the top where we walked through a guard of honour under palms and ferns with our porters singing a hymn. Glenn gave the final service where I felt emotional and at the same time felt elated, an unbelievable feeling within myself, for achieving and completing the Kokoda track.

A minibus named **AMAZINGRACE** arrived shortly after with cold drinks, sandwiches, and chicken pieces. After having something to eat and a drink we boarded the bus for a short drive to visit the Bomana War Cemetery, the largest in the Pacific with 3779 graves, 237 of them unknown Australians. For an hour we walked and viewed the white marble headstones and a rotunda of cylindrical pillows that stands on a hill behind the cemetery. It was a very moving and emotional experience. The trip by minibus to the Crowne Plaza took around 30 minutes to travel the 19 kms. After we sorted out our personal gear from the trekking gear, we said our final goodbyes to our porters. My porter, Billy, made me a Kokoda stick with my name engraved on it. I believe I would not have completed the track without his help. He was always with me and assisted me at difficult areas such as river and log crossings. I gave him some cash, 5 pairs of hike socks and gifts for his children.

In the afternoon I had a shave and a hot shower to freshen up and repacked my bags. My hike boots, gaiters and trekking poles were steam cleaned for a small charge at the hotel. In the evening we had our final farewell buffet dinner and goodbye speeches. Next morning we were up early for our flight home, leaving Port Moresby at 6.15am arriving Brisbane 9.15am.

> *I appreciate Mates4Mates very much for giving me the opportunity to walk and complete the Kokoda Track. Achieving the challenge and walking in the footsteps of heroes gave me confidence and belief in myself especially confronting my fears.*

On my return home from Kokoda I weighed myself and found I had lost 8kg (17.6 pounds). I was still suffering from dizzy spells, so I fronted my doctor. He identified I had a problem with the vestibular system in my inner ear. Apparently when I rolled down the steep slope on the Kokoda track, I had dislodged the crystals in my inner ear causing dizziness. I had an X-ray of my tail bone – coccyx – and it showed I had fractured it. My doctor said it would heal on its own and to expect to have pain for at least eight weeks.

> *The vestibular system is a part of the inner ear. It sends signals via the vestibulocochlear nerve to the areas of the brain which are involved in co-ordinating movements of your eyes and your head and maintaining balance.*

I was referred to a vestibular physio in Nambour over the next few months where I had to do vestibular rehabilitation. It involves exercises that are designed to re-calibrate the balance system, reduce dizziness and improve balance.

> *There were specific exercises such as balance and walking with a ball, head-eye coordination exercise and fitness training.*

While I was training for the Kokoda track, David got engaged to his partner Louise on September 3rd in Queenstown NZ, and just before I left for Kokoda, Michelle married her long-time partner, Neil, on the October 8th at Pelican Waters Golf Resort in the garden by the lake. Fifty-five people attended the wedding.

> *As a father I felt immensely proud of Michelle on her special day.*

On the 14th November, David and Louise experienced an earthquake of magnitude 7.8 in Wellington just after midnight

New Zealand time, and it was followed by three moderate shocks of magnitude 6.0 within twelve hours. They also experienced another earthquake on the 22nd November, registering magnitude 5.6 on the Richter scale. They were both shaken by the earthquakes and their unit was slightly damaged.

On 18th February 2017, David and Louise arrived home. They decided to quit their jobs and return to the UK and get married, but first David would have to go through the process of applying for a UK visa and marriage documents to get back into the UK. Louise departed us on the 11th April and David departed three months later, the 19th July after some frustrating moments in obtaining the correct paperwork.

In the meantime, I was chosen to attend another Mates4Mates rehabilitation challenge program, the Dawson River Retreat Trek from the 22nd to the 26th May. It was to experience the wilderness of Central Queensland near Theodore with country hospitality, bush tucker, bushman survival skills, and to canoe and trek along the amazing beautiful scenic parts of the Dawson River.

Day one:
I met up with other Mates4Mates Dawson River Retreat group members at Brisbane Airport for our 08.50am flight to Rockhampton, arriving at 10am. We were met by our guide leader, Ben, and he drove us to his property near Theodore, about a two-hour drive. After lunch we set up camp and met our other guide leaders. Travelling by a minibus in the late afternoon we visited the local Theodore Cenotaph and erected/painted an honour sign for our Australian Somali war veterans. After a service at the

Cenotaph we drove to the Dawson River and took photos. In the evening, Ben briefed us on the activities for next three days and after the barbecue, we sat around an open campfire and listened to one of our group members, Graham McLoughlin, who played his guitar, recited poems and sang country and western songs. It is a small world as I had met Graham years earlier in my working days at Rockhampton Weather Bureau.

Day two:
Started early with a barbecue breakfast. After breaky we travelled in the minibus to Isla Gorge where we walked a short distance to the lookout and viewed some amazing scenery of the surrounding country. After morning tea, we then drove to Glebe Weir and began our 14 km trek along the Dawson River towards our camp site with our day packs and water bottles. At times we had to cross obstacles, such as billabongs, fallen tree logs and push through thick grass. I was up front following our guide leader Noel who was a proud aborigine and had great knowledge of bush tucker. He pointed out and collected some small red berries from the ground and gave them to me to quench my thirst. We arrived at the camp site at 4pm where another guide, Damo, had arrived earlier and set up the campfire and caught some local fish for dinner. He had motored up the river in a tinny to the camp site with our personal gear, camping gear and some food supplies. Although tired we immediately set up our tents. In the evening we sat around the open campfire on logs and had kangaroo stew, fish and sweet damper for dinner. We chatted and listened to Graham playing his harmonica. It was a cold night and I struggled to sleep.

Day three:

After breakfast we strapped our life vests on and clambered into seven two-man canoes. At the start, the canoe trip did not go too well when one veteran went for a swim after losing his balance and falling into the river. It was difficult at first as we tried to paddle over sunken logs, snags and sandbanks. At times we had to get out of the canoes and pull them over the obstacles and along the riverbank until we got into deeper water. From there it became an easy paced journey as we passed grassy riverbanks and sandstone cliffs. Along the way to our next camp site we stopped at times to have breaks, do a spot of fishing and learn more about bush tucker. We arrived at the campsite at 3pm where Damo was waiting with the gear and again had set up the campfire. After setting up our tents we all went for a swim in the very cold and muddy water to freshen up. For dinner we sat around the crackling campfire and had chicken stew and damper. During the night I had two bad nightmares. The second one was particularly terrifying when I screamed and jumped out of my tent after hearing the sound of an explosion. I thought I was in Vietnam again in the middle of the jungle. The explosion was an actual sound from a dunny seat, abruptly closed by a veteran, who had gone to the open toilet hole. At the time his wife thought he was screaming out after falling in, but it was just me screaming from a nightmare!

Day four:

The last day on the river. Two of our group members came down with diarrhoea so Ben decided Damo, in the tinny motorboat loaded with gear, would tow the canoe with the two sick victims.

We set off in the canoes on glassy water and in misty conditions until we reached the bluff part of the river where we pulled in and some of us, including me, climbed a sandstone hill overlooking the Dawson River. The climb was difficult in spots but was well worth it as we were rewarded with magnificent views of the river and surrounding area. Descending the hill was difficult for me, slipping on loose rocks and gravel causing deep cuts and abrasions to my right knee and leg. It took us a good hour and a half to climb and descend the hill. Once down on the river edge Ben sprayed antiseptic ointment onto my injured right knee and leg. With no wind and perfect conditions, we made good progress to our final pick-up point. Back in civilisation we packed the canoes onto trailers, and then got back on the road to Ben's property. Ben's wife, Shelly, had cooked a camp-oven lamb roast dinner which was described in one word, scrumptious. After the roast dinner I enjoyed a hot shower and then we gathered around the fire and each member of the group made a farewell speech about what they gained from the Dawson River Retreat.

Day five:

I was up early at 4am and sat around the campfire until sunrise. We packed up our tents and gear, then had a hearty barbecue breakfast. After saying goodbyes, we were in the minibus back to Rockhampton Airport. We departed Rockhampton at 12.55pm and arrived in Brisbane at 2.30pm. Back to the reality of busy traffic and crowds.

> ***Although it was not as strenuous and challenging as the Kokoda track, I still had to face my challenges and fears like canoeing on the river. After my near drowning accident at***

Macquarie Island, I was scared of boating on water such as oceans and rivers. Successfully canoeing the Dawson River helped me to overcome this fear. It also gave me confidence within myself and knowledge that I could face any challenges in the future. I was also inspired by the other veterans' stories and their struggles with PTSD.

In early August I had to fly down to Victoria to do three talks on PTSD at Warragul, Hastings and Rosebud libraries.

This time I had no fear of flying, probably thanks to the recent rehab challenges.

On the 19th August I was asked by the Gallipoli Medical Research Foundation (GMRF) to attend a Media Release at the Queensland University of Technology (QUT), Kelvin Grove campus in Brisbane on **Biological Factors Contributing to PTSD**. Channel 7 wanted to interview a Vietnam veteran about PTSD, so GMRF chose me. The interview went ok and was aired on Channel 7 News that evening. QUT and GMRF released a Media Release earlier on the 17th August, including my quote. See below:-

MEDIA RELEASE

To: Sally Eeles | Executive Producer | 7 News Brisbane
Date: Thursday 17 August 2017

BIOLOGICAL FACTORS CONTRIBUTING TO PTSD

Queensland researchers find epigenetic predisposition to PTSD in war veterans and civilians exposed to urban violence

A world-first study investigating the genetics of PTSD in Vietnam veterans, conducted by QUT in collaboration with the Gallipoli Medical Research Foundation (GMRF) and funded by RSL Queensland, could help explain why some people develop posttraumatic stress disorder (PTSD) after exposure to trauma while others do not.

The findings by QUT researchers from the Institute of Health and Biomedical Innovation (IHBI) identified biomarkers which contribute to a predisposition to PTSD and can be passed down to future generations.

The study involved a cohort of 229 Australian Vietnam veterans and a civilian population exposed to urban violence from Atlanta, USA.

Recently published in the international psychiatry journal *Acta Psychiatrica Scandinavica*, this is the first study of PTSD to use the latest DNA technology to look for epigenetic changes. Epigenetics explains how environmental factors such as stress can change the way genes work without altering the DNA sequence.

"Using cutting-edge technology, we investigated epigenetic changes across the entire genome in Australian Vietnam veterans," said lead-author of the study, QUT Senior Research Fellow Dr Divya Mehta.

"We identified novel genes that had different epigenetic patterns in veterans with PTSD compared to veterans without PTSD. Importantly, we replicated these effects in a US civilian population, exposed to urban violence.

"Our results highlight that there are genes involved in the vulnerability to PTSD that are in common with neurodegenerative disorders such as Alzheimer's disease. The common mechanism in both disorders based on the genes identified might relate to tissue inflammation," Dr Mehta said.

The study is part of a wider research initiative which has revealed a number of physical co-morbidities associated with PTSD. The findings of this initiative are now being used to equip doctors and other healthcare professionals with new strategies to better identify the signs and symptoms of PTSD.

"This research is vital to shedding a light on this debilitating condition. Never before had researchers looked this deeply into PTSD and its relationship with the physical health of veterans," said Miriam Dwyer, CEO of GMRF.

The QUT research team included researcher's Dr Divya Mehta, Dr Joanne Voisey, Professor Phillip Morris and Executive Dean of Health Professor Ross Young together with national and international collaborators. This research is part of an overall $7 million research program funded by RSL Queensland.

"The more research that's conducted on PTSD, the better the chance of recovery for our veterans and also the wider community where the disease can ruin lives just as insidiously," said Stewart Cameron CSC, State President of RSL Queensland.

"This is a critical step towards addressing the physical and mental health challenges faced by those who've served our country," Mr Cameron said.

Approximately one in four Australian veterans from the Vietnam War developed PTSD. Many of these veterans were not diagnosed until decades after their service had ended. "For years I asked myself 'why me?' Some of my mates who went over there had no problems, no nightmares, no lack of sleep, no flashbacks. I could not understand why it was having such a terrible impact on me. I've had issues all my life because of PTSD," said Vietnam veteran and study participant, Dave Morgan.

"I got involved in this study to find answers, not just for me, but for everyone who suffers from PTSD. I am so grateful for this research, and that it will help increase understanding of what I went through."

END OF MEDIA RELEASE

On the 6th September Deb and I flew to London to attend David and Louise's wedding (Michelle and Neil flew into London a couple days later). They were married on the 16th September at All Saint's Church, East Sheen at 12.30pm, followed by a reception at The Royal Mid Surrey Golf Club, Richmond. About 50 people attended the wedding.

Once again, I was a proud father.

David obtained work with a European Engineering Firm in London that specializes in tunnels. He is currently working on the High-speed Rail Project from London to Birmingham while Louise is a music teacher.

We left UK on the 21st September and flew to Helena, Montana to visit Ron and Sandy. After a week in Helena we flew home, taking forty hours to arrive in Caloundra. Michelle and Neil toured Europe for two weeks before they came home.

On the 30th November I recorded a bad nightmare. It had been 58 days since I last had one, a record. All the rehab challenges I had participated in had done wonders and calmed me down.

In early April 2018 I was invited to do a talk at the University of the Third Age Rockhampton U3A, on my published books and PTSD. 145 people attended, mainly retired members of the community and I sold over 30 books. We also took the opportunity to inspect our house at Yeppoon and came away disappointed as the house was untidy and the garden overgrown. I had a go at the Real Estate Agent for not looking after my property properly. About two weeks later, I got a phone call from the Real Estate Agent telling me my house was damaged by fire. The cause of the fire was from a cigarette when a kid downstairs was smoking in bed and fell asleep. The kid survived but ended up in hospital with smoke inhalation. The whole house downstairs was gutted by fire while upstairs was smoke damaged.

It was a frustrating year in 2018 with ongoing dramas and issues with the Yeppoon house and my health but the biggest disappointment was we could not get away on holidays. We were continuously answering calls from the Insurance Company and tradespeople on issues renovating the house. One call from the insurance company triggered my **anxiety and anger**, when they informed me a tradie had accidently left a tap on with the plug in the bath for a whole weekend causing water damage upstairs and downstairs.

My health was another concern when I had a blood clot in my left leg and had to be put on blood thinners and again after having my yearly blood test, they discovered my PSA – Prostate-specific antigen levels high so I was referred to a Specialist. He sent me for an MRI scan – Magnetic Resonance Imaging and it showed I had an enlarged prostate but no cancer. The scan also showed I had a lesion in the right superior pubic ramus adjacent to a previous fracture site. For further investigation I went for a bone scan with radioactive substance injected and from the scan it showed the lesion was a fracture that had healed by itself. I believe this fracture occurred in my fall on the Kokoda track.

I volunteered to work at the Caloundra RSL Military Display Museum every Tuesday from 10am to 2pm. My rehabilitation challenges and library talks had given me self-belief and confidence in getting out and meeting people instead of isolating myself at home. When I returned from the Vietnam war, the RSL – Returned and Services League – snubbed me and most Vietnam veterans. For years I refused to go into an RSL Club because of what they did to me and other veterans. One strategy I learnt from the PTSD programs I attended **was not to dwell in the past, look towards the future and be positive**.

I am also involved in Water Quality Monitoring for Maroochy Water-watch. I had taken over the volunteer job from my daughter, Michelle, back in 2011 while living in Palmwoods.

Every month I monitor the water quality at Hunchy creek near Palmwoods. From a road bridge, I collect the water by lowering a bucket attached to a rope into the creek, then pull the bucket up. I place a Horiba U-52 multi-probe analyser into the bucket of water and record the parameter measurements of pH (power of hydrogen or potential for hydrogen), Conductivity, Salinity, Turbidity, Dissolved Oxygen and Temperature.

> ***With my voluntary work, attending gym sessions twice a week, house chores, mowing the lawn and food shopping, I found my lifestyle was busy and I was finally coping with PTSD symptoms quite well.***

My psychiatrist Dr Cadzow wanted me to attend an outpatient day program on Anxiety for ten weeks and a Trauma Recovery Program for PTSD for twelve weeks at the Cooinda Mental Health Service, Sunshine Coast Private Hospital, Buderim. After some deep thinking I decided to attend the two programs, mainly because I had gained an understanding of and ways to cope with my PTSD from previous programs. From the 8th January 2019 to the 19th March I attended the Anxiety program every Tuesday from 8.45am to 3.15pm and commuted by taxi to every session.

What is Anxiety? Anxiety is the common cold of mental health and is normal. Most people will experience some level of anxiety on a regular basis. For some people anxiety persists, escalates and has a problematic, negative impact on their thoughts, feelings and behaviour. The wide range of symptoms include feelings of panic, rapid heart rate, nausea, stomach pain, headaches, difficulty concentrating and avoiding situations.

With my anxiety/PTSD, I experience four categories of symptoms:

One: I re-live and experience my traumatic event repeatedly through visual flashbacks during the day and night, especially at night with my nightmares.

Two: I avoid anything that can trigger my traumatic event, like avoidance of memories, feelings, thoughts, and situations that are associated with the event.

Three: I have negative beliefs such as, the world is a dangerous place and people cannot be trusted. I also have negative emotions with numbness, irritability, guilt, and anger.

Four: I am hyper-aroused and easily startled.

On the ten-week program, along with eleven other participants I was introduced to **CBT – Cognitive Behavioural Therapy** and learnt helpful strategies to cope with anxiety.

Cognitive Behavioural Therapy assists in identifying and challenging unhelpful thoughts, beliefs, attitudes and to learn practical self-help strategies. These strategies are designed to bring positive changes.

We practised **Arousal Management Techniques** over the course of the program, such as Progressive Muscle Relaxation, Guided Imagery Meditation, Aerobic Exercise, Isometric Exercises, Mindfulness and Controlled breathing.

Progressive Muscle Relaxation (PMR) is a technique for reducing muscle tension from head to toes. Sit in a comfortable position in your seat, hands resting on your lap, your eyes open or closed, breathe slowly through your nose, silently counting to three and then out through your mouth again for three. Progressively tense for ten seconds and relax for 20 seconds various muscles groups from the head to the toes including face, shoulders, arms, chest, hands, stomach, legs and feet.

Guided Imagery Meditation is a natural mind-body technique that often manifests in visual pictures or mental images in our mind. Sit in a comfortable seat, breathe in through your nose counting silently to three and then breathe out through your mouth counting silently to three again, then when feeling relaxed, picture yourself in a place of relaxation. For me it was the beach and I used all my senses imagining I was there.

Aerobic Exercise is also known as 'cardio' and it involves any physical exercise of light to moderate intensity, like jogging, swimming, cycling and walking. It can reduce the body's stress hormones like cortisol and adrenalin whilst stimulating the body's feel-good hormones like endorphins.

Isometric Exercises involves the tensing and relaxing of muscles. We were told with each exercise to tense over a period of **seven seconds** and then slowly release the tension over another **seven seconds**. Some isometric exercises we were shown were:-

Cross your legs at the ankles, press and hold the tension, then slowly release.

Place your hands behind your head and lock your fingers together, press and hold the tension then slowly release.

Cup your hands together and try to pull them apart, hold the tension and slowly release.

Hold your hands palm to palm, press to hold the tension and slowly release.

Tighten your buttock muscles while sitting in a chair, hold the tension and slowly release.

Place your hands under the side of your chair and pull up, hold and slowly release.

Mindfulness can be described as the practice of paying attention in the present moment, aware of where you are and what you are doing, and not overly reactive or overwhelmed by what is going on. Typical mindfulness activities include:- Mindful with non-judgment and awareness of breath, body, feelings, emotions and thoughts. You can be seated, walking, standing or moving. It is also possible to lie down but that often leads to sleep. Mindfulness reduces stress, increases focus, increases empathy and respect, understanding of others, overcomes challenges and improves physical well-being.

Controlled breathing exercises can help you relax. Deep breathing is one of the best ways to lower stress in the body. When you breathe deeply, it sends a message to your brain to calm down and relax. Take a long slow breath in through your nose, hold your breath to the count of three. Exhale slowly through pursed lips while you relax muscles in your face, jaw, shoulders and stomach.

These techniques have been found to be beneficial in treating PTSD Anxiety. I found they assisted in calming my body and reversing the stress response. These were the main key treatment strategies I found helpful from the ten-week Anxiety program.

While I was still attending the Anxiety program, I had to attend two interviews to be assessed by a clinical team psychologist to see if I was suitable for their upcoming Trauma Recovery Program for PTSD. I found both interviews extremely dramatic for me as I had to go through my trauma in every detail, like my feelings and my five common senses at the time. I broke down on both occasions.

Note: I do not recall any of the following incident:

A couple days after the last interview, on Saturday 2nd March, Deb found me lying on my bed confused and not aware of my surroundings. Deb also noticed my left eye was closed and I was unable to open it. She immediately called the ambulance. I was rushed to the Sunshine Coast University Hospital suspecting I had a stroke. I first recall lying in bed, busting for a leak in the Emergency Ward with Deb, Michelle and Neil at my bedside. Over the next few hours, I had scans and x-rays to my head to see if it was a stroke. That night they put me into a private room and gave me some Aspirin. It was a bad night for me with a throbbing headache and I could not sleep. Next morning the Doctor visited me and said he believed it was not a stroke but maybe a severe nerve reaction. Later in the morning I was discharged, and Neil drove me home.

> ***At this stage, my left eye was opening and closing, continuously twitching. The most common causes of eyelid twitching are stress, fatigue and caffeine.***

I commenced the Trauma Recovery Program on the 26th March. The intensive program was held every Tuesday, Wednesday and Thursday from 9am to 3pm for twelve consecutive weeks. There were seven of us on the program with five males and two females, all from a Military background except for two former police officers. We were given the nickname the 'Magnificent 7', probably because we all got on well together. The program covered topics such as anxiety, depression, anger, addiction, sleep disorders and the impact it has on people with PTSD. The main aim of the program was to learn strategies to help you to relax when anxious, to confront your trauma memories so your thoughts and images of the trauma event are not so distressing and to learn ways to stop avoiding activities or places.

Every morning we had a therapy session where we sat around in a group facing our clinical team of psychiatrists and each one of us had to give a brief talk on how we were going, our feelings and our current SUDS. **SUDS – Subjective Units of Distress Scale is a scale for measuring your distress, fear, anxiety or discomfort on a scale of zero to ten**. For the first six weeks most of the group including me had breakdowns when talking about our present condition or our past journeys with PTSD. On the group therapy session my SUDS were mainly between five to eight.

Zero *is totally relaxed;*

One *is alert and awake and concentrating well;*

Two *is minimal anxiety and distress;*

Three *is mild anxiety and distress, no interference with performance;*

Four, Five and Six *are moderate anxiety and distress, being uncomfortable but able to perform;*

Seven *is quite anxious and distressed, interfering with performance;*

Eight *is very anxious and distressed, can't concentrate;*

***Nine** is extremely anxious and distressed; and*

***Ten** is the highest distress, fear, and anxiety discomfort that you can feel.*

I was also receiving weekly individual Imaginal Exposure therapy sessions with my psychiatrist, Sally, where I would sit comfortably in a chair and close my eyes and describe my trauma memory of the pit hole incident in Vietnam. Here I would describe in present tense what I saw, heard, smelt, tasted and touched when my pit hole collapsed on top of me from an enemy mortar shell. At first my SUDS rating was at the highest scale of Ten when describing the vivid memory of my trauma, but after a month my SUDS dropped to around Four with moderate anxiety and distress. At times during the sessions Sally reminded me to control my breathing and reassured me I'd be okay. At the end of each session I would practise controlled breathing and isometric exercises to calm me down.

After a month of Imaginal Exposure therapy my SUDS dropped, and I had reduced my anxiety when reliving my trauma in the exposure sessions. I then began the next stage guided by Sally in doing In-Vivo Exposure where I was exposed to my biggest fear of confined spaces such as getting into a lift. The goal of In-Vivo Exposure for me was to learn how to cope with and overcome my extreme fear of confined spaces and to act in a non-phobic way.

The first exposure, getting into the main hospital lift did not go down too well. I only lasted a couple seconds in the crowded lift when I had a major panic-attack and flash-back where I felt the whole lift was collapsing around me. I could not breathe, and felt I was choking in my pit hole again and became totally disorientated and confused where I was. I vaguely remember Sally reassuring and comforting me that I was ok, and to take big breaths and ground myself but apart from that I cannot recall what happened after I got out of the elevator.

My memory was a total blank until I found myself sitting in the lounge room with Deb by my side. I had arrived home by taxi where the taxi driver and Deb assisted me into the house. Deb noticed I was not with it, confused and could hardly walk.

> ***Memory loss is a by-product of stress and various other anxiety symptoms like panic, hyperventilation, sweating, trembling and fatigue. The main cause of memory loss is a hormone known as cortisol, released during stress.***

After the incident my family wanted me to quit the program but I felt I should continue as my doctor had warned me before I commenced the course, I would experience distressing moments like that and I asked myself why quit, as I only had a further six weeks to go to complete the program. For the next six weeks I took small steps towards my graded exposure goal of getting into a lift and staying there for at least ten minutes. While I had some minor panic attacks, I finally accomplished this goal in the last week of the program.

All seven of us on the program had similar avoidant behaviour issues like:- avoiding distressing memories or thoughts; avoiding distressing feelings, including bodily sensations; avoiding people; avoiding places; avoiding conversations that arouse distressing memories; avoiding activities; avoiding objects; avoiding situations.

During the twelve-week program, the seven of us were taken to locations to confront our individual avoidant behaviours. In mid-April we visited the Moolooaba Surf Club where I had that major flashback during the 2013 New Year fireworks celebrations. Again, I struggled as we sat in the club chatting and having cups of coffee. My SUDS was up to around Eight, very anxious and distressed, could not concentrate and kept scanning the area for danger.

I think my memory of the 2013 New Year's flashback did not help me.

Our next exposure trip was to the Big Top Centre at Maroochydore in early May for ten-pin bowling. None of my cohort members knew I was once an excellent ten-pin bowler with a couple of trophies in the cabinet and I did not let on. I used to go bowling in my Army days before I was posted to Vietnam and later when I lived in Gladstone with the Bureau of Meteorology. I gave ten-pin bowling away while in Gladstone after I had a flashback when the sounds of the bowling balls hit the synthetic lane and the impact of the balls scattering the pins. All these sounds reminded me of the different fire explosions while in Vietnam. On entry to the Centre my SUDS was about Eight and Sally reminded me to apply controlled breathing and grounding techniques to reduce the anxiety. This worked and as the game progressed my SUDS started to drop to about Three. After all the years not playing ten-pin bowling, I soon discovered I had not lost any of my skills as I won the contest. As we left the Big Top Centre all my fellow Cohort members started joking that I had tricked them into thinking that I was not much good at the game.

Our final exposure trip was in late May when we visited the largest shopping centre on the Sunshine Coast, the Sunshine Plaza at Maroochydore for the morning. Although I was alert all the time, my SUDS was on a low scale of about Three as I walked through the Plaza with two other cohort members. I think the reason for the low scale was I had visited the Plaza on a few occasions in the past.

We covered a lot of strategies on the twelve-week program and I believe I learnt a great deal about how to manage my PTSD symptoms especially my **anger** and **sleep**. Some examples of situations that can trigger my anger in **external factors** are:

Frustrations: being stuck or cut off in traffic and someone sounding their car horn at me.

Annoyances: people smoking near me, inconsiderate noisy neighbours and neighbours who fail to trim their trees.

Abuse: when people are rude, abusive and show no respect to me.

Injustice or Unfairness: sexual assault victims, crimes that go unpunished, corruption and enrichment of politicians, discrimination against the disabled, the millions of people who are affected by war and the list goes on. *This is the reason why my Doctor keeps saying to me "Do not watch television, Dave".*

Then there are the **internal factors**, such as **our thinking, our interpretation of the situation that determines our feelings**, like being late yourself or others being late, personal space, poor service, disorganisation, disruptions to schedule, being let down by others, being lied to, challenges to your opinions or beliefs and incompetence. My military training instilled a set of rules of discipline and beliefs that prepared me for combat so I cannot let my guard down; being late means something bad has happened, anyone could be the enemy and mistakes equal death.

I learnt practical strategies and improvements in my behavioural responses to **Anger** by taking note of **'The four Rs'**:

1. **Recognise** – look for your early warning signs of anger, increases in heart rate, breathing rate and muscle tension.
2. **Retreat** – stay calm, no sarcasm and no attacks. Try to talk sense. If that fails, suggest a discussion later after the situation calms down as getting upset will not help.
3. **Relax** – use relaxation strategies to reduce hyper-arousal and acute anxiety, to control breathing and grounding techniques.
4. **Repair** – come back and resolve the situation by addressing the issue in a calmer state of mind.

OR briefly, anger management strategies are **STOP, CALM DOWN, UNDERSTAND, and RESPOND**.

Lack of sleep and nightmares are big issues for me, and I believe the program helped me with ways of decreasing my nightmares and increasing my sleep. Nightmares are bad dreams that can cause a strong unpleasant emotional response of fear, despair and anxiety. My nightmares are full of psychological and physical terror and panic and often I awake in a state of distress and am unable to return to sleep.

On the program we learnt ways to rescript or reimagine our nightmares with different and less frightening outcomes by means of **IRT – Imagery Rehearsal Therapy.** IRT works by writing down the details of your nightmare either at the time or later and then rewrite your nightmare changing the story into a non-frightening, positive and happy ending. You rehearse the new nightmare story with the new ending by reading and studying throughout the day with the goal of reducing the frequency and intensity of these terrifying dreams.

I probably experienced around 150 nightmares a year while I was working, but since then my nightmares have slowly dropped and I believe the reason is because I have attended ongoing counselling sessions and PTSD programs. In 2012 my doctor asked me to record every nightmare I was having. Here are the number of nightmares I have had over the following years:- 2012 – 67 nightmares; 2013 – 69; 2014 – 86; 2015 – 77; 2016 – 68; 2017 – 40; 2018 – 38; 2019 – 32; 2020 – 25; 2021 – 24.

After waking from nightmares it would take at least an hour for me to settle down and I was always reluctant to go back to sleep because I was afraid of having another one. Often to distract myself from the upsetting emotions, I would splash cold water on my face, have a cold drink of water and either watch something on television or listen to music to calm myself down. Other techniques that assisted me at times was when I walked around the house or sat up in bed and read a book.

On the program we also covered sleep hygiene to create a sleep environment and behaviour that would improve our sleep patterns. Lifestyle factors can have a negative impact on sleep, such as caffeine, nicotine, alcohol, diet and strenuous exercise. We also learnt negative effects in our bedrooms and bedtime routines, like noise, room temperature, body temperature, air quality, lighting, mattress and pillows. We learnt to develop a bedtime wind-down routine.

We had sessions on **PTSD Depression** on the course. I have experienced severe depression on a few occasions, notably when I travelled to United States in 1975 and when I was medevaced out of Casey, Antarctica in 2004. I noticed on both occasions the less I did the more my depression worsened. A reduction or avoidance of pleasurable activities such as socialising, exercising, house chores, intimacy in my relationship and avoiding family contact and support made my depression worse.

We were introduced to **Behavioural Activation (BA)**, an effective strategy to reverse the negative impact of inactivity due to depression. Behavioural Activation is another goal of **Cognitive Behaviour Therapy (CBT)** that aims to help patients engage more often in enjoyable activities and develop or enhance problem-solving skills. You identify specific goals for the week and work toward meeting those goals.

One: You identify activities that are uniquely important to you, listing the activities from easiest to hardest.

Two: Set an action plan and identify specific goals, starting small with short-term goals.

Three: Make sure activities are specific and your progress is measurable.

Four: Continue with activities that are providing you with pleasure and achievement.

Five: Increase activities that you try to avoid.

Six: Ask friends and family members for support and help.

Seven: Slowly build up the number of activities you engage in each week.

Goals take the form of pleasurable activities that are part of the life you want to live. I want to keep fit, keep active and travel. **Note these are my weekly planned pleasure activities I would try to follow and achieve at this time**. My activities were to go to the gym three times a week, volunteer at RSL Military Museum once a week, shopping once a week, do house chores twice a week, gardening once a week, go to the RSL club to meet up with friends for lunch once a week, watch sport on television on the weekend and watch a movie at home on Saturday night.

Another practical problem solving I learnt on the program was how to curb **Depressive rumination**. I have a habit of ruminating over any problem that upsets me which causes my head to be filled with the same thoughts that just keep repeating over and over leading to depression. We were taught effective ways to break the cycle of depressive rumination.

One: Distract yourself when you realize you are starting to ruminate. Try some of your enjoyable activities such as watching television, listening to music, doing exercise or hobbies.

Two: Outline a plan of action by writing a list of possible solutions and then evaluate the pros and cons of each.

Three: Choose the most helpful and achievable solution.

Four: Carry out the plan and review the outcome.

Finally, how to change your negative thoughts and substitute them with positive ones.

One: The first steps toward changing your negative thinking patterns is understanding your thinking style. For example, if you tend to view yourself as a complete success or failure in every situation, then you are engaging in "black-and-white" thinking. Other negative thinking error patterns include catastrophising, overgeneralising, labelling, mental filtering, mind reading, personalisation blame, fortune telling and low frustration tolerance.

Two: Learn how to stop thinking negatively with a treatment plan involving Cognitive Behaviour Therapy (CBT) – cognitive restructuring. This process helps you to identify and change negative thoughts into more helpful rational or balanced responses. Cognitive restructuring involves a step-by-step process whereby negative thoughts are identified, evaluated for accuracy, and then replaced.

Step 1: Identify and become aware of your negative thoughts. Example of mind reading: "I know this bloke in the gym does not like me as he does not talk to me."

Step 2: Determine the accuracy of your negative thoughts. "Is this true?" "What proof have I got?" "How accurate are my thoughts?"

Step 3: Replace your negative thoughts with positive rational alternative thoughts. "He may be shy as he does not talk to anyone else" or "He may be concentrating on exercise."

Three: It is possible that sometimes people will critically judge you, so it is important that you are able to cope with rejection and criticism. Assertive communication involves clearly stating your opinion such as how you feel and what you want without violating the rights of others.

Four: Thought diaries can be used to change negative thinking. They help you identify negative thinking and gain a better understanding of how your thoughts cause your emotional reactions.

Five: Practice mindfulness meditation. It is the practice of detaching yourself from your thoughts and emotions and viewing them as an outside observer.

We had regular exercise sessions on the twelve-week program which I found beneficial. **Exercise** is most important for PTSD as it builds sharper memory and thinking, higher self-esteem, more energy and decreases your stress levels. We had sessions in the gym and at times on the waterfront at Alexandra Headland parade. We completed Cardiovascular/Aerobic exercise, Resistance exercise and Flexibility including stretching, Yoga and Pilates.

We also had **Relationship** sessions which wives and partners were invited to attend. Debbie did not attend these sessions because she had attended previous Relationship sessions at Greenslopes Hospital with me. I also found these sessions boring mainly because I had been through it before. I did take note of one session which made sense to me when they introduced us to **'The Sound Relationship House'** built on Trust and Commitment. Inside the house you Create Shared Meaning, Make Life Dreams Come True, Manage Conflict, The Positive Perspective, Turn Towards Instead of Away, Share Fondness and Admiration and Build Love Maps.

I also did not enjoy the **Addiction** sessions mainly because it brought back bad memories of my alcoholic days when I left the Army especially when I was in United States. I have beaten my cravings as I have not had an alcoholic drink for ten years.

The Trauma Recovery Program finished on June 13th. We had a farewell lunch a week earlier at the Mooloolaba Wharf café to celebrate the upcoming end of the program.

On June the 28th Michelle, Debbie and I flew to Perth for five days to help my older brother Gerry pack up his belongings. Gerry lost his partner, Rene, to dementia, after they had been together for thirty years. He wanted to move to Caloundra to live in a Retirement Village to be closer to me and my twin brother Don, so we arranged to purchase a unit for him at the Village on his behalf. While in Perth along with the packing, we also took the opportunity to see the sights of the city, Fremantle and catch up with my sister's family.

After we arrived back home in Caloundra, Gerry became depressed while he was waiting for the settlement date to move into the unit, and he was missing Rene as well. I also became depressed with his issues and found myself frustrated and pressured looking after his personal affairs, like going to Centrelink with him to transfer his pension to Queensland, to the solicitors about the unit and accompanying him to the doctor regarding his mental health. The day before the settlement date, he shocked us all by announcing he was not interested in living in Caloundra and he had arranged with his doctor in Perth to be admitted to a nursing home there. In the end it was a waste of time and money with his air fares, costly solicitor's fees and removalist costs. The removalist cost became even more expensive when I had to arrange for his furniture and belongings to be sent back to Perth for storage.

Gerry served in the Navy for six years when he was in his twenties and is a veteran of the Montebello Islands nuclear testing.

After Gerry flew back to Perth on the 25th July my left eye completely closed due to the stress and lack of sleep. You will remember it had started to twitch after I was admitted to the Sunshine Coast University Hospital in early March with a suspected stroke. Dr Cadzow diagnosed it as Blepharospasm caused by fatigue and stress and referred me to an Eye Specialist. The condition can be treated by toxin injections (Botox) or surgery involving the removal of eyelid muscles.

It took months before I was able to see the Eye Specialist.

Finally, in early August the renovations and repairs to our Yeppoon house were completed after it was damaged by fire in April 2018. We decided to drive up to Yeppoon to inspect the house with Michelle and Neil joining us for the three-day trip. On inspecting the house, it looked immaculately new with the bathroom and toilets modernised and the whole house painted throughout. The only disappointment was the garden and bushes outside neglected since the fire, so I contacted the Real Estate Agent to get a gardener in to tidy it up. The drive up to Yeppoon and back home was difficult and challenging, due to my closed left eye.

Debbie and I flew out to London on the 31st October for five week's holiday to visit David and Louise in their new home at Tadworth, a suburban village in Surrey in the south-east of Epsom Downs about 34 kms from London. We were intending to visit them earlier in August or September, but David wanted us to delay our trip until November as Louise was expecting their first child in late November. Most of the days were cold and miserable so we were limited in what we could do. Exercise is important for me so on most early mornings during the week I would go with David in his car to the Railway station where he would catch a train to work, and then I would walk home. Likewise, in the late afternoons I would walk to the station and meet him, and then we would drive home.

While waiting for the birth we helped around the home with cooking, cleaning and shopping to ease the pressure on Louise, but we did manage a trip to Gloucester by bus for three days to visit a cousin of mine. It was cold there with some snow and when we got back to Tadworth I came down with a bad cold – a heavy head and blocked nose – which prompted my nightmares and anxiety again.

A healthy seven pounds five ounces little baby girl named Isabella Louise Diane Morgan with bright auburn hair and blue eyes arrived in the world on Sunday the 24th November at 7.19am. It was a special moment for Debbie and me, as she was our first grandchild. On the same day Debbie and I flew to Faro in Portugal for three days to seek some warmer temperatures, on David and Louise's recommendation. It was our first visit to Portugal. Faro is the southernmost city in Portugal's famous Algarve region. On our first day we toured the city area and markets, the second day we explored the Ria Formosa Natural Park Barrier Islands of Desert Island, Farol Island and Culatra Island aboard a speedboat which was the highlight of our trip and the rest of the time we rested and enjoyed the warmer temperatures.

Although we only saw and nursed the sweet little Isabella for five days before we departed for Australia, it was better than not being able to spend any time with her. The first grandchild is a monumental moment in life as I believed I would never be able to love anything or anyone as much as my own children. It feels like I have been given a second opportunity at life and love.

What a year 2020 was. We will all remember this year as something very unusual because of the Covid-19 "pandemic". A year we will not forget, but so lucky to be living in Australia compared to other countries. From March 22nd the lockdown started with non-essential services, including pubs, clubs and restaurants, closed. Later that week, Queensland shut its borders to non-essential travellers.

With the lockdown I could not attend my gym sessions and my volunteer work at the RSL Military Museum or do water sampling at Hunchy creek. I had to cancel my annual barbecue get-together with my 104 Sig Sqn Vietnam mates, but the biggest disappointment was the cancellation of ANZAC services across the country. Many veterans like me held our own services with candles and laid wreaths at our front gates. The restrictions started to ease on May the 16th, and by June the 2nd I was back in the gym and in August commenced my volunteer work at the Museum and water sampling at Hunchy creek.

The lockdown caused a lot of mental depression for people in isolation, with generalised anxiety, irritability,

and high pessimism about the future. I found this an ideal comfortable world for me with none of the above symptoms as I was familiar and obsessed with this way of life back in my Giles and Antarctica days. It was stress-free for me with hardly any traffic on the roads, few people in shopping centres, and I did not have to attend Medical Centres for Doctor's appointments, instead using Zoom online for appointments.

In October it was all back to normal in Queensland although there were still some interstate border restrictions in place. I attended and participated in a Veteran Sleep Therapy Research Study every Wednesday from October 14th to December 9th at the Gallipoli Medical Research Foundation (GMRF) Greenslopes Hospital.

There were two younger veterans with me in the Research Study. I went by taxi to the sessions and back home. The aim of the program was to get me a better sleep and replace my nightmares with happy dreams with Cognitive Behavioural Therapy for Insomnia (CBT-I) and Imagery Rehearsal Therapy (IRT).

I have touched on both these therapy programs while I was at Cooinda hospital in 2019, but I found the GMRF study more beneficial to me especially the Imagery Rehearsal Therapy (IRT), maybe because there was a small group of us with only three veterans including me on the study program and I found our research team could concentrate more on each individual.

For over fifty years I have had nightmares, and this causes a Nightmare Cycle of more nightmares that leads to unpleasant emotions (anger, fear, etc) and disruption of sleep quality. The cycle continues to sleep impairment which leads to daytime fatigue and irritability and finally, poor coping and more stress.

With IRT, in simple words, they try to change my nightmare to a happy dream but to me it was exceedingly difficult as my trauma happened when I was asleep. It took me over a week to put one together.

First, I selected a disturbing nightmare and wrote it down on paper and kept it in the present tense. Here is one of the nightmares I wrote down:-

I am awakened by a BOOM blasting sound with my ears ringing. In darkness everything is falling on top of me. I am unable to open my eyes. I cannot breathe. I am choking. I cannot move. I am suffocating with this heavy weight on top of me. I am in my pit hole or am I in my grave hole? I feel I am in a furnace of heated hell. I am dying. Will this ever end?

After I wrote the nightmare down, I proceeded to change it into a new happy dream on paper and in present tense. Here is the new imaginative dream I wrote down:-

I am awakened from a silent beautiful restful dream on my soft bed in my safe cool bedroom breathing fresh clear air as my granddaughter Isabella jumps on top of me and smothers me with hugs and kisses and yells out "I love you, granddad."

I have been rehearsing this new dream at least once during the day for a few minutes and before I go to bed at night with my favourite music in the background and at the same time taking notice of the new thoughts, feelings and images of the happy dream. This is my new nightly routine including doing Progressive Muscle Relaxation (PMR) in bed before I go to sleep. So far it is going well.

On the Veteran Sleep Therapy Study, I wore an Actigraph wristwatch on my non-dominant wrist for seven days at the beginning and at the end of the study.

It showed I only averaged 4 hours 30 minutes of sleep time. An actigraph monitors movement and can be used to assess sleep-wake cycles.

With my left eye closed permanently due to a severe nerve reaction from the Trauma Recovery Program for PTSD at Cooinda hospital 2020, I was to attend an eye specialist on the Sunshine Coast in May, but this was cancelled due to Coronavirus. I did get in to see the eye specialist in mid-October and there is hope my left eye can be opened by Botox but first I had to have an MRI scan to my brain to assure there are no issues there causing the eye closure. The last time I had an MRI scan to the brain was in Hobart after I was medevac'd out of Casey Base Antarctica in 2004. In the MRI tunnel I had a full-blown anxiety attack and a flashback of being buried in the pit hole back in Vietnam.

This time I was prepared as Dr Cadzow gave me a script for Valium (5 mg) tablets to get me into the MRI scan tunnel. I took two tablets an hour before the scan and it worked as I cannot remember too much entering the tunnel of the scan machine. My scan results have come back with no issues to my brain so now I have to decide whether to go ahead with the temporary fix of Botox. I am not too keen.

In late November our son David, his wife Louise and their little daughter Isabella (12 months old) in UK all tested positive for Coronavirus. David was the worst with a high fever, sore throat, cough, no energy, aches and pains through his body for ten days while Louise only had mild symptoms. Little Isabella went off her food, would not sleep, had a runny nose and a slight temperature. They suspected Louise caught it from her school as a couple of teachers had come down with the virus including a class of students. Everybody at little Isabella's private Day Care Centre was tested but all were negative.

The good news is they have all recovered, although David has little taste or smell and is still fatigued. With the launch of the vaccine for Coronavirus, let us hope the world can get back to normal for 2021.

Now we are into the new year 2021, our daughter Michelle and husband Neil are expecting their first child, a little baby girl in early February. Being a grandparent is the best feeling ever as I found with our first grandchild in Isabella. Every day we try to WhatsApp David, Louise, and Isabella and seeing my granddaughter's little face melts me with joy and brings light to my day. My children are the rainbow of my life and grandchildren are the pots of gold. They are truly a gift from God and add much to my enjoyment of life.

CHAPTER 29

PSYCHOLOGICAL TREATMENTS THAT CAN ASSIST VETERANS WITH PTSD AND SLEEP PROBLEMS

Dr Sarah Hampton
Research Fellow and Clinical Psychologist,
Gallipoli Medical Research Foundation

Sleep problems are unfortunately a common occurrence among veterans with PTSD. Current figures indicate up to approximately 60 percent of ex-service personnel with PTSD have a diagnosis of insomnia (Jenkins et al., 2015; Plumb et al., 2014). This may include not being able to fall asleep, waking up repeatedly through the night, early morning waking, or not feeling rested after sleep despite adequate opportunities for sleep, which results in significant distress and/or difficulties completing normal activities during the day. Current Australian guidelines recommend the psychological approach called Cognitive-Behavioural Therapy for Insomnia (CBT-I) as the first line of treatment for insomnia (Australian Medicines Handbook, 2019). The Australasian Sleep Association (ASA) recommends that CBT-I should be used whenever possible, and medications should be limited to the lowest necessary dose and shortest duration (Grima, Bai & Mansfield, 2019).

What is CBT-I?

Cognitive-Behavioural Therapy for Insomnia (CBT-I) aims to improve overall sleep quality and quantity by addressing the underlying causes of insomnia, which are most commonly sleep thoughts (cognitions) and sleep behaviours (habits). Some examples include negative thoughts and beliefs about insomnia, spending too much/little time in bed, going to bed too early/late or rising too late, trying to control sleep, and lying awake in bed frustrated and tense. Veterans with nightmares tend to avoid bed altogether, and report many unhelpful sleep behaviours such as going to bed late, sleeping on the couch or recliner after being woken by a nightmare, and/or napping throughout the day. Self-medicating with alcohol or substances to bring on sleep is also common among veterans with nightmares.

The theory behind CBT-I is that these sleep cognitions and behaviours are learned and can therefore be *unlearned* through specific training. Some veterans report that a number of their unhelpful sleep habits were learned throughout their military service; for example, being trained to survive on very little sleep, to "expect the unexpected," and to remain vigilant at night-time. CBT-I trains participants by providing education about sleep, relaxation training, stimulus control, sleep hygiene, sleep efficiency training (also called sleep restriction), and cognitive therapy strategies.

How can CBT-I be beneficial?

Studies have demonstrated that CBT-I can significantly improve sleep quality and reduce the severity of insomnia, as well as improve symptoms of PTSD and depression (e.g., Ho, Chan & Tang, 2016). These positive outcomes are also found in the veteran population (DeViva et al., 2018; Alessi et al., 2016; Karlin et al., 2015). Unfortunately however, CBT-I does not completely solve the sleep problem dilemma for veterans with PTSD as it does not specifically target nightmares. This is why the Gallipoli Medical Research Foundation (GMRF) is currently investigating whether the combination of CBT-I and another approach, Imagery Rehearsal Therapy (IRT) for nightmares, may improve overall sleep outcomes for veterans with PTSD, insomnia and nightmares.

The problem of nightmares

Nightmares are a specific type of sleep problem that can be a common and distressing experience for veterans with PTSD. Nightmares are defined as extremely frightening dreams which usually involve a threat to personal survival, security or self-esteem (American Psychiatric Association, 2013). After waking up from a nightmare, the individual usually eventually becomes alert, orientated, and able to recall details of the dream, unlike sleep terrors where the individual remains asleep and has difficulty recalling the episode (American Psychiatric Association,

2013). Between 60 to 96% of veterans with PTSD experience nightmares (Pigeon et al., 2013; Levin & Nielson, 2007), with around a third (31.2%) experiencing nightmares on a weekly basis (Creamer et al., 2018).

Nightmares can contribute to insomnia by causing awakenings and disrupted sleep, anxiety and fear about going to sleep, unpleasant and disturbing emotions during sleep, and the use of substances or drugs to bring on sleep (which may disrupt the ability to experience deep, restorative sleep). Nightmares can also cause problems during the day, such as anxiety, irritability or short-temperedness, tiredness, and difficulties getting on with daily tasks. For veterans with PTSD, nightmares can make hyper-arousal and avoidance symptoms worse. Nightmares can occur occasionally, or with a pattern of frequency, such as daily, weekly or monthly. They may have new content each occurrence or have recurring themes, for example, some veterans describe their nightmares as 'replaying' aspects of their trauma experiences (like a night-time flashback). Nightmares may also develop into a chronic condition, which is considered to be at least one nightmare per week for six months or longer (American Psychiatric Association, 2013).

Traditionally, nightmares are thought to be a symptom of unprocessed trauma. For example, shortly following a trauma, nightmares may help the trauma survivor to re-live the experience and recall important details that might be meaningful or useful. Nightmares may also serve a critical survival function by motivating the trauma survivor to remain out of harm's way. Evidence-based treatment for PTSD is usually recommended as a first step to addressing ongoing nightmares, which involves resolving unprocessed trauma that may be contributing to the nightmares. However, some people report that their nightmares persist after receiving treatment for PTSD, despite experiencing improvements in some of their PTSD symptoms.

A more recent theory put forward by Krakow and Zadra (2006) suggests that it is possible to work with the chronic nightmare condition separately from PTSD treatment. The treatment approach is called Imagery Rehearsal Therapy (IRT), which focuses on the development and application of imagery skills. The reduction of nightmares is the primary treatment goal of IRT, rather than simply a potential benefit of treating trauma. Krakow's theory suggests that although nightmares may develop out of a traumatic experience, they can become *stuck like a broken record* that our brains have learned to replay over and over again. For example, a veteran with trauma may experience a PTSD trigger during the day, which can set off the 'broken record' at night. IRT aims to fix the broken record through the learning and application of imagery skills, with the goal to reduce the frequency and distressing nature of the nightmare(s).

What is IRT?

Imagery Rehearsal Therapy (IRT) aims to reduce, or completely eliminate, the frequency and/or distress-intensity of nightmares by using the skill of imagery to change their content (Krakow & Zadra, 2006). IRT may be delivered individually with a psychologist or mental health practitioner, or in a group-based setting. IRT first involves selecting a recurring nightmare (or nightmares with a recurring theme) to work on during treatment. The content of the nightmare is briefly written out, and then the patient is encouraged to think about how to 'rescript' the ending in any way that feels right for them (as little or as much as they wish) so that they feel comfortable, competent and in control, and with a sense of safety and/or closure. Re-scripting the nightmare does not have to be realistic – in fact, the more creative and detailed the new ending is, the more effective the re-scripting can be. For example, a patient might choose to "zoom out" and find they are in a training seminar discussing a made up scenario. Or they might decide to have superpowers that make them invisible to the enemy, or have a special ability to turn an offender into a friendly dog. However, some people prefer to make more realistic changes, like changing the weather or adding in more support. For patients who experience dreams that replay past traumas (like a night-time flashback), it may be helpful to add in reminders that the patient is actually asleep and dreaming; for example, changing the dream so that the patient is wearing pyjamas. Research also seems to suggest that making less violent changes to the nightmare is helpful (e.g., Harb, Thompson, Ross & Cook, 2012). The goal of the treatment is to change the night-time dream experience, not to alter actual real-life memories.

The patient is instructed to write out this new dream and rehearse the re-scripted dream by reading over it and imagining it in their mind before they go to sleep. It is important that the new dream starts the same way as the old nightmare, but the patient makes changes to the dream at a point that feels right to them – typically before the dream becomes distressing. This way when their mind starts playing the old broken record nightmare, it can be trained to go down a different track with the new dream that is rehearsed. Some IRT approaches may ask the patient to select their most distressing nightmare to work with first, while others may encourage them to choose the least distressing, and work towards the most distressing nightmare gradually over time.

Some veterans may be hesitant to engage with IRT because they are concerned it will disrespect or trivialise the serious and potentially traumatic life events that led to their nightmares. This is not at all the intention of IRT. The treatment does not aim to, nor have the ability to, erase, manipulate or alter actual memories of real-life events. In addition, whilst IRT uses creativity and imagination in the therapeutic process, this is not for the purpose of minimising or trivialising the trauma. Rather, IRT uses creative imagery as an intentional, specific tool in order to help the patient master distressing images experienced in their nightmares.

How can IRT be beneficial?

Imagery Rehearsal Therapy has been shown to improve sleep quality, reduce the frequency and intensity of nightmares, and improve PTSD symptoms (e.g., Casement & Swanson, 2012). IRT is thought to work in a number of ways.

Firstly, it is believed that by rehearsing the rescripted dream we are creating a 'new-dream memory', and repeated rehearsal of this new-dream increases the likelihood that when the nightmare occurs the new-dream content will be drawn from memory instead of the original nightmare content.

Secondly, Krakow and Zadra (2006) use the analogy of a metamorphosis change process; as the individual progresses through IRT, their nightmare content may naturally change to become more symbolic before eventually completely phasing out. At the same time, the emotions they experience during the nightmare, such as fear and helplessness, tend to become less intense and ultimately resolve.

Thirdly, IRT is thought to reduce the intensity and frequency of nightmares by exposing patients to the difficult parts of the nightmare and increasing their sense of confidence that they can cope. Exposure to the nightmare content (e.g., by briefly writing out the nightmare) with the support of a psychologist can reduce its distressing nature and help the patient feel more empowered. A final important aspect of how IRT is believed to operate is by changing the relationship patients have with their nightmares. It is possible that the process of repeatedly imagining the rescripted dream helps patients to feel more in control of the images that appear in their dreams. Patients tend to experience a shift from feeling powerless to feeling powerful in their nightmares, and report experiencing confidence and mastery through a proactive approach to confronting their nightmares.

Obstructive Sleep Apnoea (OSA)

For veterans with PTSD, Obstructive Sleep Apnoea (OSA) is also a common cause of insomnia. For example, the presence of OSA has been found in up to 83% Vietnam veterans with PTSD (Kinoshita et al., 2012). OSA is characterised as recurrent collapses of the upper airway resulting in reductions in airflow and breathing difficulties whilst sleeping. OSA can contribute to insomnia by causing frequent awakenings and disrupted poorer quality sleep. Some common symptoms of OSA include snoring, tossing and turning throughout the night, difficulties breathing during the night, waking up gasping for air and feeling fatigued and irritable during the day (Sleep Health Foundation, 2021).

PTSD and OSA often go hand in hand. For example, a patient may wake up in a distressed, breathless state and is unsure whether this was due to an apnoea that has triggered a PTSD-related flashback or memory, or whether this was due to a PTSD-related nightmare, flashback or memory that has triggered a state of panicked breathlessness. Phelps et al. (2018) have suggested that nightmares may be triggered by the arousal (e.g., breathing difficulties or restless legs) associated with an underlying sleep disorder such as OSA. This arousal may also make it more likely the veteran with PTSD will recall dreams (Phelps et al., 2018). It is crucial that OSA is properly assessed and diagnosed by a sleep specialist, so the right course of treatment can be determined (e.g., continuous positive airways pressure; CPAP), and overall sleep quality can improve.

How to get help

If you are currently experiencing poor sleep, nightmares, or psychological distress it is important to speak to your health provider such as your GP, psychologist, or psychiatrist. Inquire about a referral to a sleep treatment program such as CBT-I and/or IRT. If you are concerned about potential OSA symptoms, make sure you discuss your concerns with your health provider and ask for a referral for an OSA assessment by a sleep specialist. Your health provider may also be able to provide you with some information and support on how to improve your sleep prior to commencing these specialist sleep treatments, for example:

- Reducing behaviours (e.g., daytime napping and stimulating activities around bed like clock watching, TV and electronic devices) and substances known to negatively impact sleep (e.g., alcohol, nicotine, or caffeine);
- Learning relaxation exercises (e.g., Progressive Muscle Relaxation) to promote restfulness before bed-time and help with returning to sleep after awakening; and
- Establishing daily routines conducive to restful sleep (e.g., regular bed-time and wake-time schedule, increasing physical activity and optimizing day/night light exposure).

References

Alessi, C., Martin, J. L., Fiorentino, L., Fung, C. H., Dzierzewski, J. M., Rodriguez Tapia, J. C., ... & Mitchell, M. N. (2016). Cognitive behavioral therapy for insomnia in older veterans using non-clinician sleep coaches: randomized controlled trial. *Journal of the American Geriatrics Society*, *64*(9), 1830-1838.

American Psychiatric Association. (2013). *Diagnostic and statistical manual of mental disorders* (5th ed.). Arlington, VA: Author.

Australian Medicines Handbook. (2019). Adelaide. Australian Medicines Handbook Pty Ltd.

Casement, M. D., & Swanson, L. M. (2012). A meta-analysis of imagery rehearsal for post-trauma nightmares: effects on nightmare frequency, sleep quality, and posttraumatic stress. *Clinical psychology review, 32*(6), 566-574.

Creamer, J. L., Brock, M. S., Matsangas, P., Motamedi, V., & Mysliwiec, V. (2018). Nightmares in United States military personnel with sleep disturbances. *Journal of Clinical Sleep Medicine, 14*(3), 419-426.

DeViva, J. C., McCarthy, E., Bieu, R. K., Santoro, G. M., Rinaldi, A., Gehrman, P., & Kulas, J. (2018). Group cognitive-behavioral therapy for insomnia delivered to veterans with posttraumatic stress disorder receiving residential treatment is associated with improvements in sleep independent of changes in posttraumatic stress disorder. *Traumatology, 24*(4), 293.

Grima, N. A., Bei, B., & Mansfield, D. (2019). Insomnia Management. *Australian Journal of General Practice, 48(4).* Accessed at: https://www1.racgp.org.au/ajgp/2019/april/insomnia-management

Ho, F. Y. Y., Chan, C. S., & Tang, K. N. S. (2016). Cognitive-behavioural therapy for sleep disturbances in treating posttraumatic stress disorder symptoms: a meta-analysis of randomized controlled trials. *Clinical psychology review, 43*, 90-102.

Jenkins, M. M., Colvonen, P. J., Norman, S. B., Afari, N., Allard, C. B., & Drummond, S. P. (2015). Prevalence and mental health correlates of insomnia in first-encounter veterans with and without military sexual trauma. *Sleep, 38*(10), 1547-1554.

Karlin, B. E., Trockel, M., Spira, A. P., Taylor, C. B., & Manber, R. (2015). National evaluation of the effectiveness of cognitive behavioral therapy for insomnia among older versus younger veterans. *International Journal of Geriatric Psychiatry, 30*(3), 308-315.

Kinoshita, L. M., Yesavage, J. A., Noda, A., et al. (2012). Modeling the effects of obstructive sleep apnea and hypertension in Vietnam veterans with PTSD. *Sleep Breath, 16,* 1201-1209.

Krakow, B., & Zadra, A. (2006). Clinical management of chronic nightmares: imagery rehearsal therapy. *Behavioral sleep medicine, 4*(1), 45-70.

Levin, R., & Nielsen, T. A. (2007). Disturbed dreaming, posttraumatic stress disorder, and affect distress: a review and neurocognitive model. *Psychological bulletin, 133*(3), 482.

Phelps, A. et al. (2018). An ambulatory polysomnography study of the post-traumatic nightmares of Post-Traumatic Stress Disorder. *Sleep, 41(1),* 1-9.

Pigeon, W. R., Campbell, C. E., Possemato, K., & Ouimette, P. (2013). Longitudinal relationships of insomnia, nightmares, and PTSD severity in recent combat veterans. *Journal of psychosomatic research, 75*(6), 546-550.

Plumb, T. R., Peachey, J. T., & Zelman, D. C. (2014). Sleep disturbance is common among service members and veterans of Operations Enduring Freedom and Iraqi Freedom. *Psychological services, 11*(2), 209.

CHAPTER 30

WHERE TO NOW

I am one of the lucky veterans to successfully maintain a close relationship with my family. Debbie, Michelle and David have all suffered because of my PTSD. I feel for them, given what they have endured with my nightmares, depression, anger outbursts, and mood swings.

I am aware how overprotective I was while Michelle and David were growing up. Because of my reaction to dangers in Vietnam, I became suspicious and overly conscious of their safety. Out of control with my own emotions, I took control of their lives without understanding their emotions and feelings. When they left home, they both struggled with life in the big wide world and became confused and angry partly because of the boundaries I had created during their upbringing. They both now have successful lives and have dealt with the challenges they faced. The stress of war affects most veterans' children.

My unpredictable moods and abusive outbursts have also affected my relationships with my siblings. Though I was close to my twin brother growing up, Don followed different paths to me. He was more patient and academic than me, worked hard and has done well, forging a reputation as a physicist, educator and award-winning inventor. A few years back I verbally abused him and his family, something I sincerely regret to this day but thankfully we have reconciled and we speak once a week by mobile.

Life can be cruel at times. It certainly did not do me or my siblings any favours when we lost our father, but I suppose that is the luck of the draw. Don and I never knew what it was like to have a father. All we have are a few photos and stories of Dad told to us by Mum and our older siblings. However, life gave us a wonderful mother. Deep inside me, I know we were more than lucky and blessed to have her in our lives for so long.

I was in denial of my PTSD until my return to Australia following my accident in Antarctica. I had been diagnosed on several occasions by different doctors, but each time I heard the term, I stubbornly refused to listen and follow their advice. I must thank Casey Base for breaking my need for isolation, forcing me to stop running and face my fears.

Life has certainly dealt me a tough hand, as it has other veterans, but I would not swap my life. I am happy with what I have got and what I have achieved. PTSD is part of me and will not go away. It can only be modified and managed.

Bit by bit, I am healing. Part of this comes from professional help, medication, self-care, exercise, breathing, mindfulness and exposure therapy but the biggest part comes from the love and belief of my family and friends.

I will cope

GROWING UP WITH A FATHER WHO HAS PTSD AND HOW PTSD AFFECTED ME

MICHELLE McCABE

I grew up in a household where my father suffered Post Traumatic Stress Disorder (PTSD). I strongly believe my father's PTSD has had an effect on me throughout all those years growing up and now into my adult life. PTSD affects not only the one living with it, but also the family of the sufferer.

Looking back at my childhood I have very fond memories. My parents loved us, cared for and supported us as much as they could. We were fortunate to have everything and went on many family holidays together. We never went without. While I like to focus on the happy and positive times whilst growing up, the reality is, that growing up in a household with a father who was a Vietnam veteran was not an easy road and there were times when underlying issues due to PTSD would emerge.

My dad didn't talk much about his experience in Vietnam while I was young. It wasn't until later in life when he had sought professional help for PTSD that he decided to open up a bit more and tell his personal account of the Vietnam war and dealing with the illness through his book.

I had a strict and disciplined upbringing. My dad was the main disciplinarian. There were household rules to follow and if I crossed the boundary I would be told off. I would always try to do the right thing as I was scared dad would get angry if I misbehaved. I found him to be short tempered at times. Small trivial things could potentially trigger his temper. In my childhood I believe I suffered nervousness, anxiety and lack of confidence because I felt on edge at times about how my dad would react in different situations. I felt he might get irritated by things I would do or say.

Throughout the years he exhibited an impatient nature. I found him to have limited patience or time to help out with school work or things in general. My mum helped us a lot with our school work. I recall the time when dad was teaching me how to tell the time on a clock. He would easily get agitated, quick tempered and impatient if I got things wrong or couldn't understand quickly enough. Despite his impatience, he still had an interest in our education and had high expectations for us. He instilled in my brother and me the belief that getting a good education was important and to aim high. Both my brother and I attended a private college during secondary school and went on to university.

I found that during my childhood, dad didn't like going out to social events. He openly said that he didn't like crowds of people and tried to avoid those situations. He would prefer to keep to himself or if he did socialise it would be with people he already knew, like Vietnam veteran mates and people from work. Dad wasn't interested in attending my school formal or other school events. I cannot remember him going to many events throughout my schooling like parent/teacher interviews.

During my high school years my dad did some stints away from home with his work. These ranged between 6-12 months away. They were difficult times for my family. I could not fathom why he would want to work away at remote locations for long periods of time and I would think to myself *don't you care enough about your family to stay around?* I admire my mum for her strong will, love and acceptance of the situation and for looking after us. While initially hard for us all, I think as a family we got so accustomed to dad being away from us that we just got on with things. At the time I understood the postings away were to further his ambitions and to help the family financially. It wasn't until I was older when dad sought treatment for his PTSD that I realised that he also sought the isolation away from society looking for a sense of peace from the traumas of Vietnam and his battle with PTSD.

An issue I found whilst growing up was dad's controlling and opinionated behaviour which no doubt is due to PTSD. He liked to be in control of situations and would express his opinion on matters quite openly. Sometimes watching the news on TV he would get agitated with different news stories and it could trigger verbal outbursts depending on the topic. I remember him sometimes saying to me if I was watching something on TV or listening to music, 'Why are you watching or listening to that rubbish?' It was as if he didn't approve of me watching a TV program or listening to music unless he liked it. The controlling behaviour upset me and made me feel like I was doing something wrong. Rather than being supportive and accepting of my interests and allowing me to be an individual I was made to feel guilty in a way. For me, it felt like dad didn't understand or realise that we are all unique individuals who are not going to be like him or have the same interests.

He has always had a sensitivity to noise. This was quite evident when I was young. Because he was a shift worker, he would work all sorts of hours and would sleep during the day depending on his shift. This meant we had to be quiet in the house. Dad was a light sleeper. He would hear the slightest noise. Even when you thought you weren't making much noise, he would still hear you and call out 'keep the noise down'. As a child it was hard at times to avoid making noise. I always felt on edge about it and uneasy. These days my dad still gets startled by any excessive or unexpected noise. I remember one New Year's Eve our family went down to watch the fireworks on the beach. The loud fireworks going off were too much for him to handle. He was distraught and shaking with fear. It was an enjoyable moment for most people, but for my dad the loud noise triggers flashbacks to Vietnam. This is a clear reminder of the effects of PTSD.

Growing up I knew my dad had sleep problems as he had ongoing nightmares. Many times, I would wake up during the night hearing a terrifying high-pitched screech or sometimes loud yelling and in response I would race into dad's room to check on him and find him sitting on the edge of the bed or on the floor shaking with fear. Seeing him in that state was always upsetting and confronting, knowing how the traumas from the Vietnam war were still profoundly etched into my dad's mind.

Over the years, I have shown symptoms of anxiety, nervousness, worry and low self-confidence which I believe have stemmed from my dad's PTSD. At school I was a quiet but conscientious student who didn't cause trouble. I feel I didn't have a lot of confidence in myself during my schooling and would be too afraid to speak up or ask questions. This could probably be attributed to the home environment and my dad's strict and regimented measures. It wasn't until I was older, mainly after I finished high school that I started to develop more confidence in myself. This may have been because I had entered a new chapter in my life after finishing school and I realised that if I wanted to get anywhere in life, I needed to grow confidence in my abilities and speak up for myself. I am satisfied that I have worked on developing more confidence in different aspects of my life like study, work, relationships and friendships.

Throughout my career as a teacher, I dealt with a lot of worry and stress which affected my emotional health. I struggled with being a teacher and was not happy with the job. I always felt stressed out dealing with students' ongoing and challenging behaviours and feared what each day would bring. I felt I had no control of the situation. Feeling helpless, pushed to breaking point and with a lack of support from management, I decided I had enough with teaching and pulled the pin on my career. My decision was no surprise to my parents – they knew I was unhappy because I used to whinge to them about my problems.

Initially, I think my dad was disappointed with my decision, but over time he learnt not to get too worked up over decisions I make and has shown support for my future endeavours.

I get anxious when flying which I find annoying as I really love to go travelling. I worry and fear the worst will happen. My heart races fast, my hands start sweating and I become restless and fidgety. The anxiety becomes exacerbated when there is turbulence. To cope with the anxiety, I try to keep my mind stimulated with activities to focus on. However, there are times when activities are not enough to suppress the anxiety and as a last resort I take medication if I find the anxiety too overwhelming to handle.

While I have learnt to manage stress and worry more effectively nowadays, there are times I still am sensitive in different situations. If someone pushes my buttons too far, I can get emotional. I believe though that being exposed to PTSD has given me a sense of strength and resilience to overcome difficult situations in my life.

As the daughter of a Vietnam veteran and a PTSD sufferer I have seen firsthand the effects of PTSD on my dad. While it has not been any easy experience living with a person who has PTSD, over the years I have acquired a much better understanding as an adult of the effects of PTSD, the toll it has had and understand why my dad is the way he is. When reflecting back on my time growing up, I am grateful for the way I was brought up in a loving and supportive household. I do believe the strict upbringing has taught me to have discipline myself, values, respect for others and self-motivation. I don't have any resentment towards my dad because of the way he brought me up or how his PTSD issues may have affected me. I know that my dad may have been harsh at times when I was growing up, but I always know he loves me and has my best interests at heart. The way my Dad is or the way he acts is not his fault. It's because he's scarred from Vietnam and he is battling PTSD that will always be there.

I have found that since my dad started receiving treatment for his PTSD, his symptoms have improved and he has learned to manage the PTSD better. These days I have found him to be more relaxed and easier to deal with. He is more calm and collected, doesn't get irritated as much, listens attentively and shows more interest in socialising. It's like he has mellowed as he has gotten older. It is great to see him actively involved in volunteering in the community and enjoying many other activities like going to the gym. While these are positive steps forward, the journey has taken time with many ups and downs and much perseverance and it has been the ongoing love, support and reassurance from our family along with professional intervention which has helped him through it all. While some underlying issues still remain and may never be resolved because they're part of the ongoing battle with PTSD, I still believe my dad has come a long way since the earlier days when I was a child.

I am proud of my dad, not only for his service in Vietnam and many other accomplishments, but I admire the great strength and determination he has shown struggling and coping with PTSD.

THE FORGOTTEN VICTIM OF PTSD: THE SON OF A VIETNAM VETERAN

DAVID MORGAN (Jnr)

Introduction

Being the son of a Vietnam Veteran has not always been easy and it has affected and changed my life in many ways. For a long time, particularly since Dad's PTSD diagnosis, the focus has always been on his mental wellbeing, his challenges, and his story. I have felt that the adverse impacts his service has had on the family and me have been overlooked. When I was asked by Dad to contribute my thoughts for this book, I was honoured and pleased to tell my story as the son of a Vietnam Veteran. I hope that my memories help family, friends and the wider community gain an understanding of the impact being a child of a veteran can have on an individual.

First becoming aware of Dad's PTSD

I was four years old in 1990 when Dad decided to march in the

Anzac Day parade for the first time in many years. This was the first time Michelle and I witnessed Dad march and it helped us gain some understanding of his service in Vietnam. Before heading down to the Anzac service Michelle and I got a photo taken with Dad wearing his two medals. We all went down to see the parade and watch Dad march with other veterans in Gladstone, Queensland.

Michelle and I were oblivious at that time of the affects that his service had on him and our family life even though we were experiencing the consequences firsthand. For as long as I remember Dad always had a strict, disciplined approach to parenting Michelle and me. He also had an explosive streak and could get angry quickly, particularly at Mum who took quite the brunt. I did not think at that age that this was in part a legacy from his Vietnam war experience and I just took it as normal. I understood he used to be in the Army and that he was a veteran of the Vietnam war but not much was said about his experiences. Vietnam was rarely talked about and I cannot recall many Vietnam vet mates visiting us in Gladstone.

The first incident that stands out during my early years that Dad had issues was one day in 1991 when Mum purchased a new 4-piece wooden dining table set for the house. It was delivered and placed in the house while Dad was at work. Upon his return home, the sight of the new dining table made him explode with anger. He shouted at Mum telling her off for buying it and said he didn't agree with the purchase, it wasn't needed, and it was a waste of money. A heated argument ensued with Mum, with her eventually breaking down crying. It was hard for Michelle and me to witness, and I was confused who I should support. Mum just wanted a nice dining set for her kitchen, that was her point of view and I could not see anything wrong with that. Dad just could not accept it. The fight went on for a while and in the end Dad refused to accept the table, and in his rage, he pushed the chairs and table out to the front patio in a rough manner and moved the old dining set back in its place. I had seen him in angry outbursts before, but this was at a new level.

There were other arguments between them during this period and several where Mum threatened to leave. In some of these arguments I was looking on or hearing them from a distance and hearing Mum threaten to leave made me sad. I wondered sometimes when Mum drove away in the car whether I would see her again. Dad was very controlling over every aspect of family life. I didn't understand a lot of these arguments, but I did know it affected Mum. We had noticed during this period that she had developed red blotches over her skin, which we now know was caused by the stress and anxiety from the arguments with Dad and his overpowering nature.

Although the arguments were not nice, they did move on from them and we were generally a happy family. It was a Jekyll and Hyde situation. Most people probably thought we were a model family with no issues as the arguments were always behind closed doors and only Michelle and I witnessed them.

I didn't understand it at the time, but Dad was silently suffering from Post-traumatic stress disorder (PTSD) caused by his experiences in the Vietnam war. It was only to be diagnosed many years later when Michelle and I were adults.

Yeppoon Years

The move to the coastal town of Yeppoon in 1993 was initially viewed as a good move for the family, although a few years into it, the pressure built up for Dad which impacted Michelle and me. With a long work commute, tiring shifts and a strained work environment, the pressures and anxiety built up in Dad.

Coming home, he had little patience or understanding for Michelle's and my schooling particularly some learning difficulties we faced. Mum provided the most help in our homework tasks, but sometimes Dad would view her soft and patient method as the wrong approach. On several occasions he would come in, take command and implement his strict teaching approach. Each time I dreaded this and wished he left me and Mum alone to work through my learning problems. It started with his lack of patience which sometimes led to frustration and anger.

I struggled at reading in my early to mid-primary school years. I recall several times Dad sitting me down on the couch and getting me to read a book from school. My reading out loud was slow and attempts at pronunciation of some words were incorrect with the odd stuttering. Dad would interject when I got something wrong and correct me, however, he quickly got frustrated with my errors and he started having a go at me for making errors and not learning as quickly as he wanted. He'd make statements in an impatient tone, like, "*this is easy … come on*" and "*I could read when I was your age*". Each statement was probably his way of encouraging me, however it was knocking my self-confidence. I then became conscious of making more mistakes that would get more statements and frustration from him. I felt terrible as I was trying my best but it was not good enough in Dad's eyes. The session ended in an argument, Dad giving up and telling Mum to teach me in a tone of helpless resignation. Unfortunately, his approach was that if he was teaching you something and you did not understand or learn it the first time then you were no good. He had no patience and did not make for a good home teacher. It made me feel like I was dumb and not living up to his expectations which were set too high.

Sports

Dad loves sport and while living in Yeppoon he encouraged me to join the local Aussie Rules and Soccer clubs. Dad was the coach of my soccer team for 3 seasons. My sporting experience was very enjoyable, however, Dad's strict and disciplined approach to life was evident in his soccer coaching. He was fair to the other players in my team, but I sometimes got the raw end of his coaching. If I was not playing well in a match or made mistakes, he would pull me aside at half time and give me a harsh 'rev up', aimed at making me fire up and get angry in the hope of improving my game, which most times succeeded. I was like a fresh army recruit receiving instructions and small insults barked at me by a drill sergeant. Mum could see this and would tell Dad to calm down and not be so harsh, but it fell on deaf ears. Even a parent of a fellow teammate thought Dad was particularly harsh on me and mentioned this to Mum. But Dad was adamant his coaching style was harmless. That was how he learnt things in his Army training.

Although I accepted Dad's 'rev ups' I felt pressured to perform consistently and when I didn't, felt I was letting him down and not meeting his expectations. Dad could not attend every match and when he didn't and it was just Mum I felt less pressured and could just enjoy the match no matter my performance.

Computer Games Noise

Like most kids growing up in the 90s, I enjoyed playing computer games, particularly shooter style games, usually by myself as Dad never played them with me. One of my favourite games had sound effects of various firearms and explosions and I enjoyed playing these sounds out load on the computer speakers. One day, not long into the start of the game, Dad burst into the living room and shouted at me to turn off the sound. In an angry tone he yelled, "*I can't stand those sounds, they sound like I'm in Vietnam!*" I had no idea this could be a problem for him. I felt upset that I had triggered some bad memories for him. I turned off the sound and only had it on when he was not home, but I was continuously conscious going forward about playing any kind of shooting sound either from a computer game or from TV. The realism was too much for him to take.

Dormant Volcano

When I was 12 years old, the first sign that I had taken on some of Dad's traits was when my Grade 7 teacher, Mrs Christiansen, nicknamed me the '*Dormant Volcano*'. She explained to Mum during a parent-teacher interview session, that she was shocked to witness me have angry explosive episodes in class usually at fellow classmates. She was shocked as I was for the most part an incredibly quiet and good student. On occasions I would explode with anger in my classroom and she saw a side of me she was not expecting. I was picked on by other boys and I could only take so much until I exploded, yelling at these boys in class. Mum knew that I had picked up my father's explosive trait although at that time Dad had not been diagnosed with PTSD. This observation of me by my schoolteacher went no further than a simple acknowledgement.

It was at this time that Dad was looking at ways to escape the pressures of the Rockhampton office and he succeeded by securing a 6-month posting to Giles, a remote weather station in the Gibson Desert of Western Australia. This posting was for staff only so Dad would be leaving the family behind in Yeppoon. He discussed it with us, but it was not something I could or wanted to stop Dad from doing. I did not fully understand at the time that it was his anxiety stemming from his PTSD that made him want to leave home and work at a remote station.

High School

Giles and the beginning of bullying

Dad's posting was to start in March 1998, within my first year at high school at St. Brendan's college, a local Catholic all boy's school. Dad's departure coincided with a week-long school camp at Waterpark Creek, Byfield National Park. I had said my goodbyes to Dad before my first day at camp, but I received a surprise visit from him on his final day at home when he visited me at the campgrounds. It was a great surprise and he brought me some chocolates and lollies as a treat. I spent a good 10 minutes with Dad before we said goodbye, hugged and he drove off. It was sad seeing him drive off, the last I would see of him for 6 months.

Bullying at school

Unfortunately, Dad's departure to Giles came at the worst possible time, as I soon started to suffer from frequent verbal and physical bullying at high school. In the first couple of years the bullying was almost a daily occurrence. I tried my best to ignore the bullies, but it affected me greatly including getting involved in fist fights and skirmishes to defend myself or to fend off the bullies. This was all happening in a Catholic Boy's school where we held morning prayers every day.

I missed Dad's support during the bullying in my first year at high school. He tried to provide support and guidance from afar, but it was not as effective as if he was home. I could not have a proper chat with him about it as phone calls to Giles were brief due to costs and at the time, we had no internet for emailing or mobile phones for texting.

For ANZAC day 1998, Dad was at Giles and he encouraged me to march, wearing his medals, in the Yeppoon parade. I retrieved them from his room – they were in a small box within an old brown envelope. The memories came back of the story he told me bitterly, of how he received his medals by post and had never been presented with them on parade on RTA. I joined my school in the parade and was given the honour of leading the school at the head of the march along with two other boys who had medals from relatives. I felt very proud to march with Dad's medals although sad that he was away.

Michelle, Mum and I did experience some sense of freedom around the house while he was at Giles. Free from his dominating presence around the house, we could watch what we wanted on TV and did not have to be quiet as mice in the house because of his nightshifts and fear of triggering a nightmare. However, there was a wonderful reunion at the airport on Dad's return in September. We went to Daydream Island in the Whitsundays for a holiday and settled back as a complete family unit again.

Even with Dad back and his correspondence with St Brendan's Administrators, the bullying at school continued. I started to become despondent with school. Meanwhile, Dad did not enjoy his return to Rockhampton Met office and started investigating transfers elsewhere in Australia. In late 1998, he had floated the idea with the family of a move to Mildura in Victoria. Dad and Mum did research into the move, even contacting schools for Michelle and me to potentially attend. For weeks the move was discussed, and Dad applied for the posting and I soon felt that it would become a certainty. This brought me hope and happiness that I would be escaping the bullying at Brendan's.

In early 1999, Dad received notice that he had been selected for a Bureau posting to Mildura weather station in northwest Victoria. All he needed to do was to officially accept the posting. I desperately wanted to go to escape the bad bullying I was experiencing. Dad also wanted to go to escape the stressful office environment at the Rockhampton weather station so it seemed a sensible move. However, Mum and Michelle did not want to go. Mum was settled in Yeppoon and Michelle was to commence her penultimate year of high school which she was enjoying at St Ursula's. The family was split.

After one school day in early 1999 Dad confronted the family in the evening and told us that he had decided after considering the situation that we would not move to Mildura. It was ultimately due to significant disruption to Michelle's schooling. I was devastated and felt let down. My thoughts were on my helplessness in the face of continual bullying. That night I had a meltdown. I argued with Dad and Mum, pleading for them to reconsider the move to Mildura, but it was in vain, the decision was made, we were staying put in Yeppoon. I now hated the place and was looking forward to a new start in Victoria. I expressed my hatred for school and stormed to my room. I grabbed my new 1999 St Brendan's diary and ripped it to shreds in protest. Paper was scattered all over my room. Dad and Mum tried to console me. I eventually calmed down for the night, but I can never forget how close I came to escaping St Brendan's.

After the failed Mildura move, Dad applied for the remote Willis Island weather station off the North Queensland coast. If he could not move the family then he would do a solo move to a remote posting instead. My feelings were torn – I was excited for Dad to do this extreme posting but having had a difficult time at school while he was at Giles and with the bullying continuing in my second year of high school, I was not looking forward to Dad being away again. Dad wanted to escape his workplace and I wanted to escape the bullying from school. It was looking like only Dad would succeed in escaping home. Ultimately, I didn't oppose Dad going to Willis Island and the rest of the family also approved. Dad submitted his application and was promptly accepted for a 6 months' stint between June and December 1999.

On the final school day before Easter holidays I stupidly fractured my upper right arm. I was in a sad state from the bullying at school, a broken arm, missing the soccer season due to my fracture and Dad about to leave home. He reconsidered the Willis posting and decided to pull out which came as a surprise to me. Doing so ended his Willis aspirations, although it didn't stop him looking for other postings. This time he set sights on a prestigious one – Antarctica.

1999 was a hard year for me. The bullying had worn me down and the numerous efforts by Dad and Mum to try to get the school to stop it had little impact. I was sad and helpless at high school and I slipped into depression. 2000 was the year Dad was supposed to set off on his first Antarctica expedition, but several health setbacks stopped him from being accepted on the expeditions.

In grade 11 I received another setback when I was physically assaulted by a teacher. The assault severely upset me as did the school's attempt to sweep the incident 'under the carpet'. Boys who witnessed the assault did not want to come forward, fearing retaliation from the school and teachers. My attempts to get justice failed and all this happened just months before Dad again left the family, this time for a posting to Macquarie Island, a sub-Antarctic island, for 7 months. Dad did his best to support me before he departed and he told me for the first time that he was sexually assaulted in the Army when he was a young man. This experience had obviously affected him, and I gained a little more understanding of some of the demons Dad was facing within himself but in normal circumstances would not let the family know about. We were united in our anguish and injustice from both our assaults.

All too quickly Dad was off to Macquarie Island and it was just Mum, Michelle and I again. During this time, I started my final year of school. The time Dad was at Macquarie Island was again a hard period for me as I had to deal with mentally recovering from an assault and bullying. Phone calls with Dad were even more limited than when he was at Giles, too little time to discuss any personal issues in any detail. I became angry. I had no father figure in the house to help me. I took my frustrations and anger out on Mum, getting into arguments over little things which tipped me over the edge very easily.

Dad returned home in March 2002. His stories and adventures on Macquarie Island were inspiring to me. He had a taste for the Antarctic expedition lifestyle, which was obviously helping him with his PTSD, as it was not long before he had applied for another Antarctica expedition, this time at Davis Station Antarctica. I completed high school in late 2002 and the day I received my final scores Dad was away in Hobart awaiting his departure for Antarctica. I did very well in my final grades, unfortunately there were no celebrations. It felt hollow and overshadowed by Dad's departure for Antarctica.

Dad was very overprotective and extremely conservative in his views, to the point that I was not allowed to attend schoolie events upon completion of high school. Schoolies' week was seen as a rite of passage upon high school graduation. There was not one school mate I knew who was not going to be attending. Even the so-called nerds were going. I was so embarrassed at not going that I lied to friends when they asked if I was. I respected Dad so much that I would not dare to question his views or go against what he asked me to do. I did feel deep down that I was missing out on what was only to happen once in a lifetime, finishing school. Like many of his justifications, he linked it back to his Army experience. He would say "*why do you need to go to schoolies? When I finished school, I joined the Army!*" I knew for a long time I wouldn't be able to attend as he didn't allow Michelle to attend her schoolies' event two years earlier, despite her pleading and protests. In the end I did not attend schoolies. It was just another disappointment to end my turbulent high school years.

University years

After a challenging time at high school, I retreated within myself at University, focusing on studying my hard engineering course, with vision of a better future once completed. In 2003, Dad was again away, this time in Antarctica at Davis Station.

After his return from Davis, it came as no surprise when Dad again accepted another expedition to Casey station Antarctica in 2004. Even though it was sad to see him leave again it was not as heart wrenching as earlier expeditions. We had become accustomed to him leaving and his absence from home. We just had to get on with our own lives.

Dad's Casey expedition was cut short on his first day on base by a devastating accident. He sustained terrible head and neck injuries after slipping on ice at the station, falling backwards and hitting his head on rock-hard ice. The blow knocking him unconscious and caused bleeding on the brain and ear. Medevaced by helicopter and transported back to Australia, it was a cruel end to his Antarctic career and ultimately his work career.

The accident shook the family, and we were on edge after hearing the news until his condition improved. I had a feeling of helplessness not being able to be with him and only receiving daily updates about his recovery during his 2-week voyage to Hobart.

Dad's recovery at home was long and he slipped into depression which was hard on the family. His nightmares increased and he started to get more involved with fellow Vietnam vets and the local veteran drop-in centre. It was at this time he realised he was suffering from PTSD.

Nightmares

Dad's nightmares were always a constant occurrence while we were growing up. I noticed that as the years passed, the frequency and intensity of his nightmares increased. After he returned home from his Antarctica expeditions and following his head injury at Casey, I noticed his nightmares became worse. I would be woken by him yelling out and I knew it was a nightmare. Rushing into his bedroom, we'd find him, most occasions, on the floor shaking and still mentally in his nightmare. During some bad ones, if I turned on the light or placed my hand on him to comfort him, it would spook him even further as if he was still in his nightmare. Not even words from me could snap him out. I learnt to just stand back and wait until he snapped out of it and came back to reality. He would be shaking all over, especially his hands and was soaked in sweat. I felt helpless. I wanted to help him but could do nothing.

I remember him having bad nightmares on family holidays. The exhaustion from travel and sleeping in an unfamiliar environment were triggers. On one occasion I recalled him having a nightmare and yelling out in a scared voice repeating the words "VC". But on most occasions, his nightmare reaction was to yell and jump out of bed running which was most frightening for us. In the pitch dark and not aware, he would run into furniture, hurting himself. I would try to grab him before he seriously hurt himself. The following days would reveal bruises or cuts sustained from his clashes with furniture. The nightmares were not confined to home and hotels but there were also a few occasions on long haul flights where he would wake up yelling out to the shock of nearby passengers.

Growing up with his nightmares made me afraid of making any sound in the house that could spook him and trigger one. We had to be quiet as a mouse when he went to bed. The legacy of his nightmares is I am now a light sleeper and I also get spooked by noises. It's as if my brain is now trained to listen out for his nightmares in order to attend and help him.

It is difficult seeing him have nightmares because each one is mentally and physically affecting him, both in the short and long term.

Brisbane

Following University, I moved to Brisbane for a new start in 2009. I was hoping for a better time and more independence but unfortunately in my two years in Brisbane I found it difficult to adjust to city life and making new friends. My strict and disciplined upbringing clashed with the realities of city life. I found it difficult to see intoxicated youths looking for trouble during my train journeys home, seeing graffiti, and hearing and witnessing crime, and other issues that blight most big cities. I was sheltered from this type of world growing up in a small town. My mind was trained for strict discipline and I somehow could not ignore all these issues around me. Peers my age just ignored it and it never bothered them. I was told several times that I was too serious and acted more mature than my age. I questioned why it affected me so much and the only answer led back to Dad and my strict disciplined upbringing, taking on Dad's sometimes serious nature, and being sheltered. I blamed my struggles on my upbringing and questioned Dad about it which led to arguments.

Dad and Mum could see I was not happy and recommended I see a counsellor using the Vietnam Veterans Counselling Service (VVCS). I was stubborn and dismissed the recommendation but after having many arguments with Dad, I reached a breaking point one day in 2010. The only way they could get me to see the counsellor was to take me there and go in with me at short notice. The counsellor asked us in turns about our issues and grievances and for Mum and I it all seemed to stem from what Dad was like or did or did not do in the past. It did not take long before we all broke down. It was a stark reminder that we had all suffered adverse effects from Dad's PTSD. Dad finally realised what impact his Vietnam service had on his family's lives. Although Michelle was not present, she was impacted the same by Dad's PTSD.

The counselling sessions were helpful, and it felt good to get issues off my chest to someone outside my family. Prior to this I did not feel like anyone else would understand or properly listen to my issues, so I kept everything to myself, Dad and Mum. Most of my peers did not have a Veteran as a father and

I felt that my upbringing was so vastly different to theirs that none of them knew what I was going through.

Despite the counselling, I still struggled to cope with my life in Brisbane so I decided to get away from Australia on an overseas holiday. I travelled for 5 weeks through the USA and Canada by myself in May and June 2010. The trip was a godsend. I spent 2 weeks in Montana with Dad's American Vietnam Vet mate, Ron Casey and wife Sandy. The different environment and being outdoors skiing were what I needed. My confidence grew with the wonderful hospitality and I was astounded at how Montanans and Americans in general were fascinated to meet me. I then did further travels across USA and Canada boosting my confidence. The freedom and independence of traveling by myself was liberating. It felt like my issues in Brisbane were a world away.

I returned to Australia brimming with confidence and felt that there was nothing wrong with me, but it was my home situation and Brisbane that was the problem. Unfortunately, upon my return to work, the worst was yet to come when I experienced harassment at my QR job. This led to depression again which led to more arguments with Dad even though he was trying to help. The harassment caused anxiety and stress. I felt helpless as I went through the correct workplace channels, but the harassment continued for months and was not resolved. I reached a new low in depression and sought help from GPs. One put me on anti-depressants which was the first time I had been prescribed them. They made me numb, with a no-care attitude but I knew this was not the long-term solution and wouldn't stop the work harassment.

Leaving Australia for Canada

I never forgot how great it felt travelling the USA and Canada and how differently I was treated. I felt the only solution was to pack up and leave all my troubles behind me. I was convinced this was the only option I had to escape my depression and arguments with Dad. At the end of 2010 I applied for and received visas for Canada and UK. In early 2011 I left my QR job and took a one-way flight to USA where I would stay with Ron & Sandy before heading up to Canada.

It was an emotional goodbye to Dad, Mum and Michelle. I felt that Dad was blaming himself for my unhappiness and troubles and the reason for leaving Australia. He questioned his parenting, the first time I sensed he started to reflect on his actions.

After several weeks in Montana, I was fortunate to get an opportunity to interview for a job in Calgary, Canada just north of Montana. I landed the job and for the remainder of 2011 I lived in Calgary, making some lifelong friends along the way. It was just what I needed, a learning curve, but complete independence. Although I kept in regular contact with Dad and Mum, living in Calgary and starting everything from scratch was liberating. It wasn't without some challenges and at times questioning if it was the right move, but I thought that this was just a start and I could build on what I had achieved.

London and beyond

With one more year left on my UK visa, I looked for a job in London. Deep down inside it was really the UK and the dream of travelling Europe that was beckoning. Luckily, I was working for a large global engineering firm. At the end of 2011 I could not resist the lure of UK and applied for several engineering jobs posted internally. I was successful and the process of transferring over to the UK office seemed easy. In Dec 2011, I once again moved, this time to London. It was a great feeling working in two cities in the one year.

Things just got better when I entered a London office full of friendly young professionals keen on socialising. I eventually lived in London for the next 3 years, climbed out of depression and met a wonderful girl, Louise, who eventually became my wife.

On my return to Australia, I no longer had arguments with Dad. We had learnt our lessons and Dad was receiving regular psychology sessions to help with his PTSD. He was more understanding and was, in some part, a changed man. Dad had also noticed that I had changed for the better from living overseas and also due to Louise's influence.

Louise and I lived in Wellington, New Zealand for two years and in 2017 we married. I am now a father to a beautiful baby girl, Isabella, and the joy of having her is a constant positive influence on me.

Rehab programs

Witnessing Dad participate in various courses to help him with his PTSD has been good to see. However, it was particularly difficult to see him go through the rehabilitation program he undertook in 2019. Despite its claims that it would ultimately improve Dad's coping with PTSD and reducing his nightmares, it meant he had to openly face his darkest memories. Video calling him from the UK on a regular basis, I could see the course was taking its toll. It was difficult to see him become flat, tired and hearing him confide in me that he was not looking forward to the next scheduled rehab day each week. After each rehab day he looked exhausted and it seemed his nightmares were continuing. I thought it was not good for a 71 year-old to undergo such mentally challenging rehab, but he persisted and was stoic. One day in early March 2019 I tried to call Dad but could not get hold of him for a while. Hours later he messaged me and I video called back. I was shocked to see him in hospital, with one eye shut, having suffered a suspected stroke. A call to Mum and Michelle told me the full story. It was clear that the rehab course and the breakdowns he was encountering in the course were physically affecting him.

I felt helpless being halfway across the world and just wanted to go back to help him out. I was saddened that this experience has led him to have permanent problems with his left eye. It was at this time that my wife found out we were expecting a baby. I could not wait to tell Dad and Mum, as I knew this would lift his spirits and give him something special to look forward to. A month after his stroke, it was a wonderful moment informing him of the news and he was over the moon and incredibly happy at becoming a grandfather by the end of 2019. The news changed his complete outlook and his mental wellbeing, and he coped much better with the remainder of the course.

Transgenerational Trauma

From Dad's PTSD programmes I have learnt of the concept of transgenerational trauma, whereby the symptoms and behaviours of a person with PTSD are passed on to their children. Looking back at my childhood, it is clear to me that I have picked up many of Dad's traits both good and bad, including his explosive anger, anxiety, light sleeping, antisocial behaviour, impatience and more. I hope to minimise these bad traits in myself and by cut the transmission onto my children.

Outcomes

Dad is my best mate, and we are very close despite the challenges we have faced. No one is perfect and I know that deep down he meant the best for me. Even though we had arguments in the past, I am not angry with him. I unfortunately continue to suffer occasional negative emotions such as anxiety, stress, and anger but I continue to improve. Dad shares with me the coping strategies and best practice from his PTSD programmes to help me deal with the legacy effects of his PTSD on me.

Being the son of a Vietnam veteran has not been all negative. Some traits that Dad instilled in me such as determination, discipline, perseverance, and a sense of adventure have helped me through some tough times and helped me in my achievements in life such as obtaining an Engineering degree, forging a good career and traveling and working overseas.

I am proud of my Dad and think he has achieved a lot despite his challenges. His efforts to become a better person handling his PTSD are commendable but to write an account, for the benefit of others, about his PTSD journey and how he copes with it, is a credit to him.

THE LAST WORD

Debbie Morgan

Dave never talked about Vietnam when we first met but I discovered shortly after we married that he had issues. He had a lot of anger within himself and did not seem to trust people. He wanted everything perfect and precise. I guess this came from his time in the Army. I found he wanted a perfect wife and he was always conscious of my weight and what I should eat. He demanded the house be kept immaculately clean all the time.

He brought Michelle and David up in a disciplined way, like they were in the military.

Dave's biggest issue was sleep and nightmares. After a while I could not sleep in the same bed as him as he always grumbled that I was disturbing his sleep and scaring him by my movements in the bed. He would unmake the bed every night, untuck the sheets and blankets before he got in. His nightmares were bad. He would jump out of bed, screaming and shaking and in fact any little disturbance, like someone going to the toilet, creaking house noises or noises from outside, would set him off. The whole bed would be damp from his sweating during his sleep and nightmares. I would be always washing and eventually buying new sheets, pillow covers and pillows as they would turn yellow because of continuous dampness from his sleep and nightmares.

In the end, I believe everything got to him – his work, bosses and the community but his biggest problem was battling his demons with PTSD which led him to seek isolation.

In total Dave was away from the family for two and half years (30 months) – Giles, 7 months, Macquarie Island 7 months, Davis 15 months and Casey 1½ months and that includes training.

If he had not been medevaced out of Casey, it would have been 38 months. Looking back, it was hard on the family and maybe when Dave had his accident at Casey Base, God may have been trying to tell him something.

As a wife, along with Michelle and David, I supported Dave in wanting to leave the family for each remote posting. We had long discussions each time.

Dave believed he wanted to take up these remote postings, because firstly, it was a dream or ambition of his; secondly, it would be a financial benefit for the whole family with payment of private school fees and university fees, plus money for house improvements; and thirdly, he hated working at Rockhampton with the long drive and shift work especially the 2:30 am starts.

Overall, it was hard for us all, even for Dave. It was difficult for Michelle and David not having a dad around for advice and support especially in their challenging teen years. At that age they needed their dad more. For me it was like I had lost my husband for ever; no companion to talk to or share my feelings with; nothing, just an empty feeling.

I say the hardest times were the goodbyes with tears, then our lonely holiday breaks and weekends. Apart from sport in the winter months, we did not do much. For Michelle it was netball, for David it was soccer and for me I joined the Tourist Information Centre to work on Saturday mornings in the Centre. It just seemed we were waiting around, waiting forever until his return. We did go to Brisbane once by train to visit my family, but our holidays seemed empty or without a purpose.

Christmas was extra hard. Dave was away for two of them, at Macquarie Island 2001 and Davis 2002. Christmas is all about family, but Dave was not with us to share the joy, gifts and Christmas feast. Although we had contact by phone and email, it is not the same as in person.

A lot of people including our friends questioned why he was leaving the family all the time. Was it because he did not care anymore about his family or was he selfish and thought only about himself and his ambitions?

One lady even suggested "if it were my husband, I would have left him ages ago". Another person commented, "You and your children must be very understanding or patient to tolerate a husband and father like that."

To be honest, I started to think that way myself. Dave always grumbled it was harder for him leaving the family than for us, as he reckons we had each other. That may be so but it was Dave's final decision, not ours. We accepted his decision to make him happy, following his dreams and his obsession with isolation. If we tried to stop him, he probably would not have forgiven us.

He said he would not have stopped us if we had been in a similar situation and pursuing our dreams.

In the end, was it worth it? After Dave's accident at Casey base he was let down badly by the Bureau of Meteorology and Antarctica Division. For me, Michelle and David his accident was like a nightmare, not knowing what to do. The Bureau and Antarctica Division left us in the dark. When I received the phone call from the doctor at Casey base, it was left to me to organise our plane trip to Hobart, plus accommodation for the family with no help or assistance from the Bureau at all.

With all the stress I became ill and lost weight. It took me a couple of years to recover.

For Dave it is an ongoing event with headaches and neck pain. He paid the price for pursuing his dreams but for the first time, he acknowledged that he had mental problems with PTSD and finally sought help.

I also discovered for the first time when attending the DVA PTSD programs that I was not alone struggling with his illness as wives and families of Vietnam veterans were also living similar lifestyles and had issues like us.

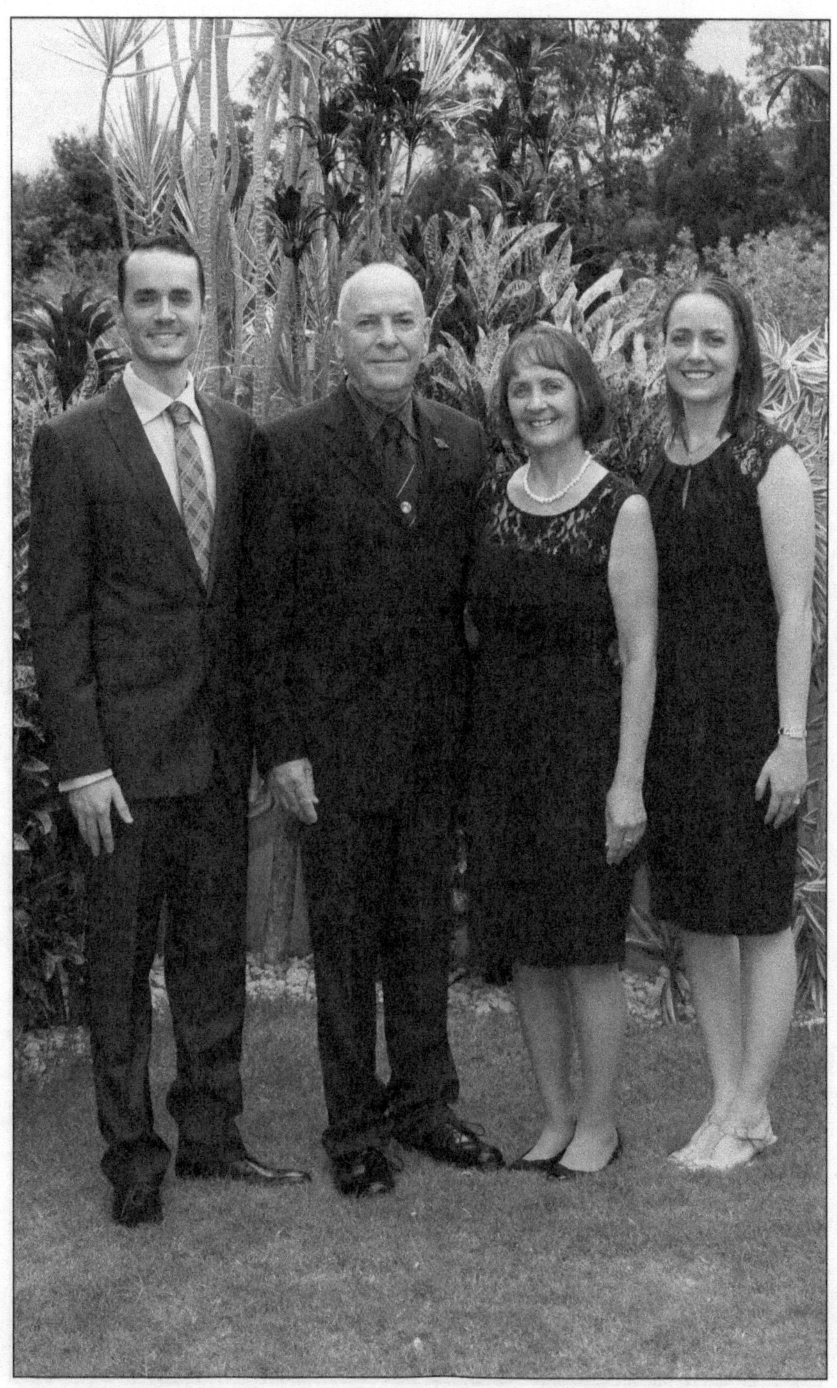

From L-R. David (Jnr), Dave, Debbie, and Michelle. Taken 2016.

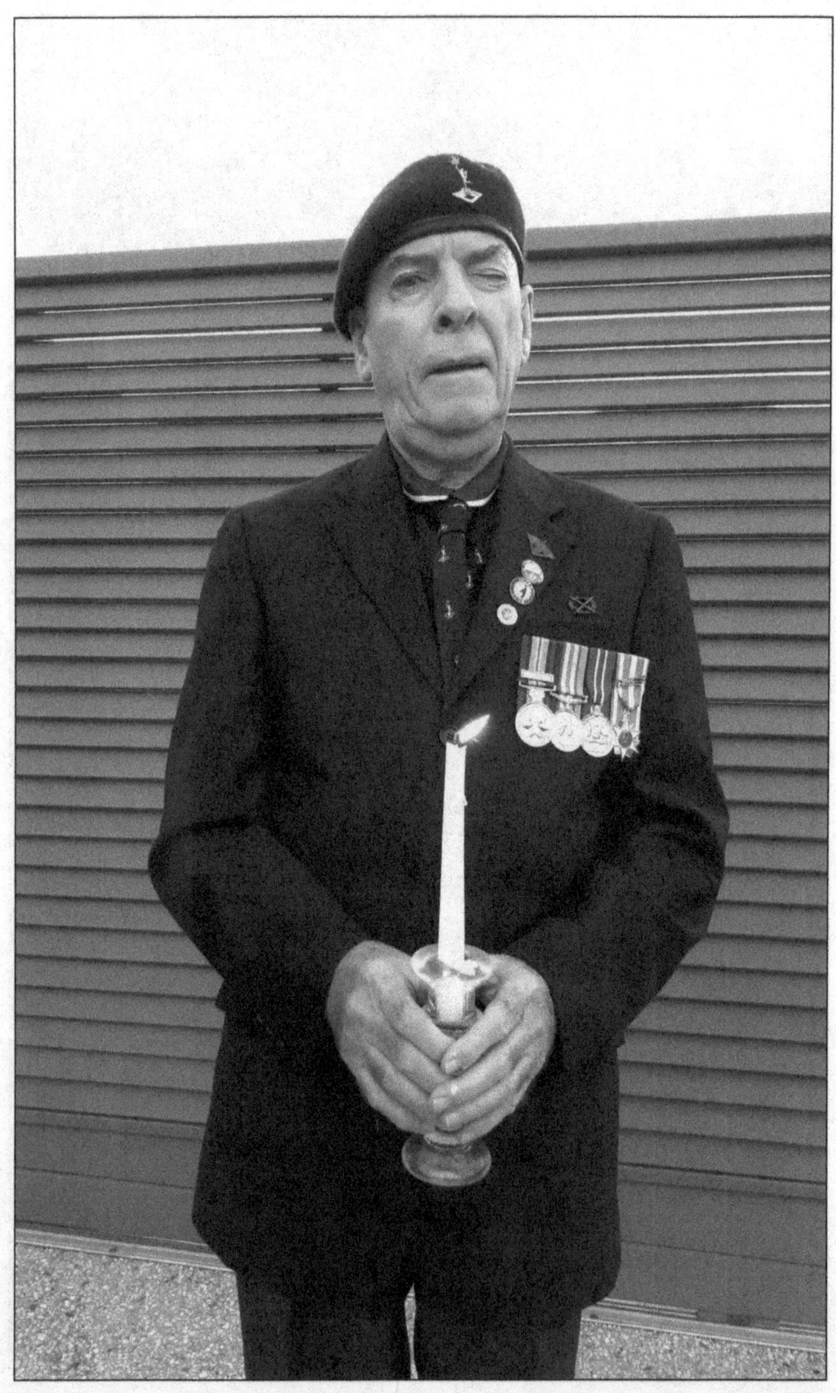

Dave at dawn service outside his house on ANZAC day 2020 (Covid restrictions).

MAUREEN BRONJES (MOZ)

Veteran

My 38 year military career was predominantly as an Investigator in the ADF Investigative Service, where I saw far too much death, crime and mistreatment of military personnel.

I loved my job. It was not a glorified career by any means, yet it meant so much to be able to see each person for who they were. So, having it cut short for health reasons was hard to come to grips with.

My life can be summed up in one simple phrase: *"Life of a Gypsy Camouflaged"* (the title of the book I'm labouring over).

PTSD became an issue late in my career and the reasons for it can be fixed to three moments in time.

The first was on a 6 months' deployment in Timor. Two Timorese were shot by our troops. I was on the scene almost immediately investigating, protected by Infantry security from a very angry, vocal crowd of young Timorese men. I was standing alone with just an unarmed civilian female Filipino investigator when I turned to see our security drive away and watched with anger as the vehicles disappeared. A sudden feeling of being surrounded came over me. In reality I was the only armed Army person left. Fear consumed my very being, a barrier I needed to push through, and do whatever needed doing to get us out of there to a safer place.

The second was in Afghanistan while investigating the death of an ADF soldier when the first vehicle of our patrol hit an IED. The patrol reacted immediately with practised drills which was reassuring.

The third moment brought home to me the fact that PTSD can affect those who love us, those who lose their heroes. At the AWM closing ceremony I was reading an account of the life of one of the fallen. There I met the soldier's son, a frail distinguished gentleman named Norman, who never saw his father again after saying goodbye, aged 10, at a train station. It was at that very reading I felt a truly honoured member of the Defence Service, which provided an opportunity for Norman to mourn his father and finally let go.

PTSD came on me through the experiences of my chosen career. Others less fortunate than me had life happen to their loved ones at a distance, but the effects are etched so deeply within them that letting go of that trauma feels almost impossible.

I am one of many who suffer the darkness deeper than anyone can know and this is why I say some of us live like a gypsy camouflaged from others.

The mirror never lies of my many days gone by

My smiles, fears and pain, ever etched on a face lined and framed

Stories of old, some problems solved

I stand before myself knowing not all is fully told

A door appears so bright and clear
Surrounded by building blocks that have shaped
Who I've become, my dear
Stepping forward with my vision strong and true
While shadows, demons and clouds slowly begin to be removed

PTSD may forever be within me, with reflections, dreams and memories now and then. Perhaps relief will come in accepting that within, we are all only human.

A COMMANDO'S FIGHT AGAINST INVISIBLE INJURIES

Andy Fermo
Afghanistan
Two Commando Alpha Company – 2007
Two Commando Bravo Company – 2009

I was born in the Philippines, the eldest of three siblings. My parents migrated to Africa for a couple of years when I was one year old, then my Dad got a job in Australia in the mining industry so I grew up in mining towns. I had to make my own fun and go out and meet new friends as we were always moving around. My formative years were full of adventure, playing with my brother, sister and mates in the backyard and the bush but as I got older, I wanted more adventure, so I joined the Army cadets. I enjoyed that, learning new skills like shooting guns, climbing and experiencing the flying fox.

This was the perfect transition from childhood to adolescent life. I eventually left the cadets when I got into the high school years and succumbed to the party lifestyle, grew my hair long, played the guitar, went to surf parties. Girls were the order of the day. I was still pushing the boundaries when I graduated from high school, but I wanted to do something more serious with my life that my parents would be pleased with. I loved music and my greatest ambition at the time was to build my own amplifier. University was not for me, so I went to TAFE (Technical and Further Education) and completed an Electronics Engineering course. I fulfilled my ambition by building my amplifier which I still have to this day. I was still partying hard and sort of lost my way through lack of motivation but with a little bit of an epiphany and intervention from my family and friends I ended up joining the Army, signing up as a Reservist.

Once I was back into the Army lifestyle at Kapooka, I sort of found myself again and with my adventure desires rekindled, I decided to go full time and get a trade. I fronted my section leader about a trade where I could use my technical skills and at the same time be in infantry-style stuff and be able to shoot a gun in the field. He suggested EW – Electronic Warfare where I would get to play sneaky-peeky stuff and go out with the infantry guys plus jump out of planes, but the job came with a top-secret clearance. I signed up for the trade and after gaining that top-secret clearance I attended the communications school where I enjoyed learning my new trade. After graduating, I was posted to 7 Signals Regt at Cabarlah in Queensland in signals electronic warfare.

Soon afterwards I was attached to 3 RAR doing some man-packing stuff, radio reconnaissance and jumping out of planes. A couple of years later I was posted to 4 RAR and shortly after, when Australia hosted the Commonwealth Games in 2006, I found myself helping and supporting the SF – Special Forces in domestic counter-terrorism in Perth. It felt to me like a whole new adventure seeing these guys practising their mission profiles, doing preparation training by jumping out of helicopters with flares going off and the sounds of gunfire. This was my introduction to the Special Forces commandos, and it was bloody awesome.

I was desperate to get a bit of that action, so I fronted the boss and it was a simple process putting in the paperwork for the Special Force Commando selection. The selection process was a gruelling program where I was pushed to the limit. I am not a tall bloke, not the fastest and not the strongest but I have got self-determination. I am only five foot six inches (167 centimetres) compared to some big blokes built like brick shithouses, well over six foot (183 centimetres). Out of the 120 soldiers who started the intense selection process only about 30 got through to the next stage and by the end of the gruelling, daunting final test, only 20 were selected to graduate as special forces commandos – including me – to wear the coveted "Sherwood Green" beret with pride.

I felt so proud of my achievement especially being the first qualified commando within my trade. Shortly afterwards in 2007 I was deployed to Afghanistan and the realisation set in that this was the real thing.

For the next six months I always remained hyper-vigilant, living fear became normal with bombs going off, the sound of machine guns and bullets whizzing past. In battle I trusted the guy next to me and I was especially lucky as I worked with a

Commander who demonstrated the best leadership qualities that I have ever met. Everyone would follow him, and he was the type of leader that everyone could talk to. With his authority he would bring out our best, whether as a team or as an individual.

I reached the pinnacle of my career when I was awarded a commendation by Special Operations Commander, Major General Hindmarsh for my tireless work and highest order of achievements on my first tour of Afghanistan. I felt good.

My second tour in 2009 was a bit different from the first, a different team and company but still some amazing people. On our first mission which lasted a month we had a few casualties. The first one was a good mate of mine Sergeant Brett Till, who was killed by an IED – improvised explosive device – when he was dismantling it. It was terribly sad, and I did not get a chance to process what happened as within a few days, we were in series of contacts and our team ran over a big roadside bomb which blew up our vehicle. Lucky for me I was in the back so although I got injured, my injuries were not as bad as those of the men in the front. A lot of the guys got traumatic brain injuries from the impact.

Those IED incidents were starting to become far too common so they decided to make use of our helicopter capability because there was often one predictable way in and one way out of most places by vehicle. There were a lot of traumatic events and near misses on that second tour, but I had to put them to the back of my mind to deal with later because I had to be operationally focused. I was there on a mission to look after our EW – callsign, the platoon, the company and the mission.

When I got back home, I was a different person, very disconnected. I started partying hard, drinking heaps with my mates. Alcohol and prescription type meds abuse became my way of coping. I was trying to decompress in my own way, but I clearly did not know how to do that properly so I self-referred to an organisation called Open Arms, to a psychologist. I wanted to check in to see how I was but at the same time not to commit career suicide by saying I was not quite right within myself. I did not want the Army to know because I was so focussed on continuing with my platoon's exciting commando stuff. The Defence Force's zero tolerance with drugs, discipline and mental issues forced me to keep my problems to myself which I think was my undoing. I admitted some issues to my reviewing officer and said I had self-referred to a psychologist but they were resolved.

For me, honesty is the best policy, so I thought the interview went well. I was meant to go to the USA on some tasking but on the morning of departure, I get a call to report to the boss who told me I had lost my security clearance because of my problems. Suddenly, I found myself barred from the highly secure area, restricted to the Q store issuing mobile phones. I felt angry and felt the system had turned on me and let me down. I had no more purpose. My skills were useless, from a top-secret clearance to an unclassified job. I was worthless and I had great fear about my future which exacerbated my symptoms of PTSD.

What was making my PTSD worse was the fact that I got separated from the military before I had the chance to finish playing soldier. I believed there were at least another two or three

Afghanistan trips in me, as some of the other guys I knew who stayed in that little bit longer got another two or three trips in.

I was medically discharged in April 2010, but it felt like a shameful discharge as I was shut off from all opportunities to continue the career that I loved. All up I did almost ten years, discharged only a month before my long service leave. They could not even leave it that one month so I could get my entitlement – another hard pill to swallow. The only positive for me was I was dating my girlfriend now wife, Claire, who I married in October 2010 and she was like an immovable rock. She supported me even though I had become aggressive, frustrated and angry, often lashing out at her.

Within two days of my discharge I found a job as a mature age apprentice chef at one of the top restaurants in Sydney. I slowly went downhill over a period of a year, and probably at my lowest point, I was trying to decide what my next job would be. Claire told me that I needed to sort myself out and even my mate Mick from Afghanistan pushed me, telling me to deal with my problems, sort myself out and get my claims in.

This I did, I set out a plan and looked for some support services. The first important step was going to my local RSL sub-branch to engage an advocate. I was fortunate he was a great advocate, a Vietnam veteran, who understood what I was going through. He taught me the tools to work on my self-care and guided me through my claims with the Department of Veterans Affairs – DVA. I will always be grateful to him as he cared about me, was willing to go in to bat for me, and was able to give me the most important and crucial advice about getting the right care. I had a great baseline.

My mental health support system in Sydney was excellent – my counsellor at Open Arms (formerly VVCS, Vietnam Veteran's Counselling Service) and a psychiatrist.

I completed an intensive outpatient program learning some invaluable tools. I learnt self-care using exercise, breathing, mindfulness, trauma exposure therapy, and CBT (Cognitive behavioural therapy) programs. I did everything that they told me to do and the program gave me a sense of purpose. I continued to be counselled for some time and after Claire fell pregnant, we decided to move somewhere quieter, so we shifted to Wagstaff on the southern part of the Central Coast just north of Sydney. It is a beautiful spot. There, I started an online property business, selling property and helping people who were affected by the global financial crisis. The business gave me a purpose again.

The good times didn't last long. In 2013 I spiralled down to rock bottom again. I stopped doing all those things I enjoyed, things like music. All my PTSD symptoms started coming back to me, nightmares, anger, etc. During the slump Claire surprised me by giving me a new paddleboard. This inspired me to set new goals. I competed in the world's most challenging paddle race, Molokai 2 Oahu, a gruelling fifty-two-kilometre race between the two Hawaiian Islands. I completed that quite emotionally but with a deep sense of self-fulfilment.

We moved up to Noosa on the Sunshine Coast Queensland in 2016 because we were kind of priced out of the housing market due to the Sydney housing boom and to be closer to our kids' Nana. As much it was the best move for us, it was challenging.

I had a great support system in Sydney, but I found Noosa had less resources. There were so many veterans up on the Sunshine

Coast and so few doctors accepting Veterans Affairs type stuff. With no support system in place to rely on, I spiralled down quickly, going off the rails again with my PTSD symptoms, nightmares and anger coming back. It took me a good 18 months to find a GP and a Psychiatrist. I finally found support and managed to start getting out of the hole again and I thought I was in a good position working hard after resuming my business in the property industry.

At the end of 2018 I had another major setback after we attempted to secure a loan to buy a home. It was the time of the banking royal commission. I had been saving for a while, but the bank believed I did not have a sound income to repay the loan. They said I needed to go and get a job to increase my income, so I closed up my old business and got a paid job which I did not really like, finding work for other people. I went into work overdrive, neglected my self-care and tried to do my best for the sake of my family. I was soon back in the hole that was even darker and deeper, when the loan fell through unexpectedly. I lost everything – the deposit and the house – to try to satisfy the bank's requirements. In the end I only had my wife and kids and family support.

For Christmas 2018 we were homeless, so we went camping at a place called Kilkivan near Gympie to lick our wounds and that is when the idea of 'Invisible Injuries' came up. I said to my wife Claire, *I need to get my issues and myself sorted out* and Claire suggested I start journaling and writing down my dreams and goals and share my story with others. This what I did, and soon found I was getting out of that dark hole and becoming positive. I was invited to speak at different events such as 'Stories of HOPE Australia', and 'Conversations' in Noosa to share my story. It felt great speaking at these events and I realised it might be possible to help other veterans and first responders with PTSD by sharing my story.

I have spent all of 2019 trying to map out my 'Invisible Injuries' vision. I got a writer and strategist on board to develop my vision and I am trying to build relationships with other ex-service organisations like Young Veterans and be more involved with my local Tewantin/Noosa RSL sub-branch. 'Invisible Injuries' is giving me a lot of purpose and it is important for me. It's aimed at creating awareness and positive conversation around the condition of PTSD and hopefully improve the lives of sufferers and their families. It's also about connecting people to the right support services.

Music has always been a big part of my life. I learnt to play the guitar as a teenager and love Rock 'n Roll, alternative type sounds and discovered dance music so I started my own DJ (disc jockey) business called DJ Antix Noosa.

This DJ business was my saving grace after I started going off the rails. Now I entertain many people on a weekly basis at corporate events, product launches, milestone, birthdays, the occasional wedding and all those types of gigs. I really enjoy being able to put my DJ Antics hat on and share my love for music and help people. I have done some gigs at Veterans Retreat. Sharing music with veterans there has proved to be a great equaliser, an ice breaker in terms of breaking down the stigma of talking about personal problems, especially PTSD. Sharing mindfulness mixed with music programs with friends and our key audience on our social media network is also important to me.

I am also focused on getting funding for a documentary and building the website. We have raised money for that and have some key collaborators coming in to sharing great information through varied programs for the benefit of veterans and first responders.

Lastly, we are planning on heading off in late February 2021, starting off in Southeast Queensland for a twelve month's national awareness campaign on 'Invisible Injuries'. This will include mindfulness through music and stuff like that. We are working with a filmmaker to document our tour and outline our approach to mental health. My main aim is to spread the word about PTSD, mental health and ways to go about recovery.

Web: invisibleinjuries.org,au
Facebook: www.facebook.com/invisibleinjuriesaustralia and www.facebook.com/djantixnoosa
Email: invisibleinjuriesaustralia@gmail.com

IMPACT

Ian Fraser

Airfield Defence Flight of Number 2 Squadron Royal Australian Air Force (2 Sqn RAAF) Phang Rang Republic of Vietnam

Introduction

Because of recent Psychiatric reports connected with my current request for an increase in disability pension and the associated Administrative Appeals Tribunal (AAT), I undertook a soul-searching review of my constant aggressive behaviour patterns.

With the assistance and guidance of my psychologist Ms Hannah Lupo I began to realise that my aggressive behaviour was a learnt negative behaviour to suppress my underlying fear of not trusting people.

As a child and teenager, I was easy-going and had lots of friends and meaningful relationships. This was despite both of my parents, who served during the Second World War, being heavy drinkers. They became very ill in my late childhood and early teens. (My father had a heart attack and subsequent stroke in the early sixties and my mother acquired kidney and liver disease and died whilst I was in Vietnam).

This easy-going personality changed early in my period of active service. I lost trust in other people and organizations. I avoided dealing with these issues by becoming task orientated and managed any interpersonal relationship problems with aggressive behaviour.

I now accept that seeking to sustain such avoidance strategy requires substantial effort. Furthermore I would like to both think of myself, and be known, as a caring person. I have always been honest except in recognizing that my negatively reinforced behaviour has prevented me from taking advantage of the many important and rewarding opportunities that have come my way.

Therefore, one purpose of this document is to signify my acceptance of my Experiential Avoidance condition[4] and commit myself to ongoing therapy to normalize my condition and to live a meaningful and rewarding life.

Background

Enlistment and Training

I enlisted in the Royal Australian Air Force (RAAF) on the 18th of February 1969 as an Air Force Defence Guard Trainee (ADG T). I first completed Basic Training, which was not specialised ground defence or infantry training, but rather an induction course into the RAAF.

4 broadly defined as any attempt to avoid uncomfortable thoughts, feelings, memories, images and physical sensations—even when doing so creates harm.

Following that initial training I then undertook my specialist trade training at No 3 Aircraft Depot from 13 May 69 to 11 August 69 at the Defence Ground Defence Training Flight.

At the end of the course I was posted to the Ground Defence Flight of Base Squadron RAAF Base Fairbairn ACT. During my period with the Flight I received no specialist training for a deployment to a war Zone. This was in stark comparison to Army personnel who attended a Jungle Training Course and intensive pre-deployment training, the kind of training my brother, Edward (who was in Vietnam when I arrived there) received from the Royal Australian Army. Indeed, a significant part of my duties in Canberra was my participation in Ceremonial Duties. I did attend one exercise in Darwin in January 1970; however, the exercise was not designed around what was happening in Vietnam and demonstrated to me how little emphasis the RAAF at the time put into Ground Defence.

Number 2 Squadron Phang Rang

In March 1970 I was posted to the Airfield Defence Flight of Number 2 Squadron Royal Australian Air Force (2Sqn RAAF) Phang Rang Air Force Republic of Vietnam. I neither received nor undertook any pre-deployment training or briefings on my role, operations or even the unit I was posted to. Upon arrival at Phang Rang I did not receive any in-country familiarization training or briefings. I arrived one day and on the next participated in my first day patrol outside the perimeter of the base.

No 2 SQN was a bomber unit flying Canberra Jet Bombers and was under the operational control of United States Air Force (USAF) 35th Tactical Air Wing (35 TAW) and was based at the

USAF Base Phang Rang in the then Republic of South Vietnam. The primary task of the Squadron was offensive bombing operations in the Republic against North Vietnamese Army (NVA) and Vietcong (VC) targets inside South Vietnam.

The Squadron was made up of around 270 personal including aircrew, aircraft maintenance personnel and support personnel. The support personnel included Administrative staff, Supply Staff (Supply, Catering and Transport) and Security personnel. Our Flight was the major part of the security section.

The Security element of the Squadron was made up of RAAF Police and Airfield Defence Guards. There were thirty-three members of the Airfield Defence Flight, an Officer, a Senior Non-Commissioned Officer (Flight Sergeant) and three sections of ten airmen commanded by a Corporal.

There were around seventeen thousand USAF, Korean, American Army, American civilian and Australian Air Force personnel. The base covered a significant area and the perimeter was more than seventeen kilometres long.

The base was under constant rocket and mortar attacks and in February there was a ground attack by North Vietnamese Special Forces (Sappers). In my 377 days at the base, it was hit by rockets on 177 occasions.

Role of the Airfield Defence Flight

The members of the Airfield Defence Flight undertook the following tasks on a six-day rotation:

- Night Patrols outside the base perimeter to set up listening/ambush positions up to 1.5 kilometers from the perimeter.

- Day patrols outside the perimeter of the base in our area of operations.
- Escort duties for vehicles leaving the base for civil affairs activities, supply and medical trips to Cam Ran Bay and escorting personnel to the recreation facility located on the South China Sea.
- Acting as an observer in Forward Aircraft Controller (FAC) aircraft.
- Acting as a Quick Reaction ground force for the RAAF Domestic Area, Flight Line and to support the Section on Night Patrol.
- Any other operational task outside the Base such as Securing downed aircraft and guarding the recreational facility at night-time in conjunction with USAF personal.
- Building and maintaining Bomb Shelters and defence sites around the Domestic Area and 2 Squadron's flight line operations.

The breakdown of the six-day cycle was two days of Night Operations, two days on standby and two days on day patrol or daylight activities. During the two day standby we were often recalled for duties such as escort and other activities.

Apart from the continual rocketing of the base, the most dangerous and stressful duty was the night patrols.

Usually we had dinner at between four and five and prepared for the night operation. Just before dark we kitted up with our weapons and made our way to the Base Security Headquarters complex where our Corporal received a briefing. We then proceeded to the section of the perimeter after dark, exited the base and patrolled to our ambush listening post. At around four o'clock in the morning, we patrolled back to the perimeter and re-entered the base through the fence just around dawn.

1. Incident on the 8th of June 1970

We departed for an ambush site just outside the perimeter on the 7th of June. On arrival at the site, we were split into two groups around the two machine guns we were carrying. The position was close to the Airfield Landing lights which extended outside the perimeter. The position was on a paddy field bund and the two elements of the section were separated by a rock formation. The machine gun in the forward group was pointing left and my gun, which was located on top of a rock, pointed right.

Just after midnight, the evening was shattered by gunfire and screams. I could hear my mates in the first group screaming and see the flash of enemy fire. As I had no way of knowing if any of my mates were dead or wounded, I began firing my machine gun over their position towards the enemy. The enemy then concentrated fire upon me, and numerous bullets passed just over my head. At that exact time an American aircraft began landing at the Base. The runway lights came on and the plane flew through my exchange with the enemy. For many years I felt that I had hit the plane, however, I now believe that it was hit by enemy bullets which were aimed at me.

I turned to my Corporal to get instructions on what to do next, however, he was frozen with fear. After I and several other members commenced shouting at him, he reacted. He called in mortar illumination and sought advice from the base. Several of our group saw the enemy retreating from the site to our left and requested that we engage them. However, instructions from the base prevented this action.

We then took stock of our casualties: one member was wounded, and another had the weapon shot out of his hand.

We retreated from the site and occupied a position around a hundred meters to the rear. We returned at dawn to determine if there was any sign of enemy wounded or dead.

Review of the Action

On return to the base we discussed the incident. What happened was that the person who was supposed to be on the machine gun went under the cover of a ground sheet to light a cigarette. Unfortunately for him that was the precise time the enemy entered the position. Only one person in that group was alert – the one lighting the cigarette – and no one else was manning a weapon. Once the firing started, they did respond. The one lighting the cigarette ducked – an action which saved his life. He was hit by two bullets and narrowly missed by three which struck a rock just above his back. The machine gunner attempted to raise his weapon however it was knocked from his hands by a bullet strike which damaged the weapon. A third member of the group rose to engage the enemy, however he had illegally altered his rifle to fire on automatic and the force of the weapon being fired on full auto knocked him onto his back so his shots went harmlessly up into the air.

Obviously, the fact that a member of the section had compromised our position by lighting a cigarette was not mentioned to the Flight Headquarters. Doing so would have resulted in disciplinary action for both the Corporal and the airman concerned.

There was never a detailed debriefing of the action by our Officer or Senior Non-commissioned officers. I did however, later meet the pilot whose plane had been hit!

Impact on me

As a non-smoker I felt betrayed by the action of the person who had compromised our position. His effectiveness was destroyed and for the remainder of his tour he was carried by us. Unfortunately, smoking during these night ambushes was allowed by the Corporal which was against all principles of night operations. Consequently, after this and subsequent patrols, I lost confidence in his leadership capabilities. Also, as I had counselled the airman about altering his weapon prior to the action I was mad at him for doing such a stupid thing. I believed that I was the only one who took the most effective action and nearly paid for this with my life.

I developed a view that I was better in combat than my colleagues. I began to question the safety of our operations and decided to become the Forward Scout to ensure if we clashed with the enemy again, I would be solely responsible for my safety.

Because of the perceived lack of leadership and support from our Officer and Senior Non-commissioned officer and the Air Force in general, I quickly became a problem airman who responded aggressively when I felt threatened. I lost most of my respect for authority. However, because I never perceived my actions as a weakness, I never sought advice from my superiors about changing my attitude. This was the start of my avoidance problems with authority. If I did not trust my superiors, I discounted any advice that they could provide.

Another problem with the Air Force at the time is that we were regarded as tradesmen rather than combat personal. We were regarded in the same light as aircraft technicians, cooks, supply, and administration airman. A 'them and us' mentality developed, so much so, that even today, fifty years after the war, Airfield Defence Guards are the only mustering that marches in Anzac parades. I have never attended a 2 Squadron reunion!

A comparison of my personal reports from before and after the incident indicates how I was beginning to change.

In May 1970, my annual assessment read that I was:

> 'an average Airman who requires more time in his mustering in order to improve his professional knowledge and its application, He is far too young in his mustering to even consider his potential as an NCO. Unlikely at this time.'

However, after the incident my annual assessment in February 1971 read as follows:

> 'An ADG whose dependability has always been doubtful and who always has an excuse for obvious misdemeanours. It is unlikely he will ever reach the standards for NCO consideration.'

Whilst this assessment was correct in assessing my attitude. I strived to be the best Forward Scout I could be, and this showed through in several difficult situations the Section was involved with. Furthermore, during several other incidents, my skill levels became more advanced which increased my belief in my own abilities.

2. Incident during a subsequent Night Patrol

The next incident occurred in the same area as the first contact with the VC. By this time, I was the Forward Scout of the Section. We were moving towards our ambush position. I heard noise in front of our patrol. I stopped the patrol and we adopted a defensive position. I was ordered to advance on my own to check out the source of the noise. During the reconnaissance, I saw a person lying under an ox cart some forty meters in front of our line of advance. My Corporal instructed me to advance over the open ground to investigate the person and to kill them if they were hostile. The section covered my movements over open moonlit ground. As you can imagine I honestly believed that I would be killed as I approached the position. Upon arrival at the cart, I discovered the person was asleep with his head facing towards our approach.

I placed my left hand over his mouth and was just about to plunge my combat knife into his chest when he woke but could not scream because of my hand over his mouth. He went into complete shock and went limp as he thought I was going to kill him! His terrified face with his eyes sunk into his skull was immediately seared into my consciousness. I still have the vision of this poor man and it has been the source of countless nightmares over the years. Luckily in the split second before I would have killed him, I noticed other Vietnamese nationals to my left hidden by trees. In my earlier approach I could not see these people.

While I held the man down by lying upon him with my left hand holding the knife across his throat and using him as a human shield, I trained my M16 assault rifle (the weapon was capable of discharging 20 rounds in 1.6 seconds) in my right hand towards the other people. Had the man resisted, I would have killed him and opened fire on the group!

Moreover, if that happened, my section would have also opened fire to defend me. The Corporal this time had arranged fire support so I strongly believe a massacre would have occurred.

However, after I called out to the other people in broken Vietnamese to raise their hands, they quickly responded to my orders, and I called my section forward to support me, which they did, surrounding the group. We then discovered that they were harvesting rice in the moonlight. However, as we were in a free fire zone, they could have all be killed!

We searched them for weapons and were instructed by our base to order them to return to their village. After escorting them there, we retired.

As a result of this incident I could not sleep properly for decades. Indeed, I only learnt to handle the disturbing thoughts while attending a PTSD course in late 2016.

Unfortunately, at the time and for decades afterwards this incident had a profound effect on my personality. I wrongly believed, that if a person was not prepared to do what I had done that night they were somehow substandard. Not surprisingly, as most people do not experience this, the vast majority failed my distorted test.

Furthermore, I had learnt what it was like to go awfully close to violently killing another human being at close quarters. I would use this hard lesson from that day on to convince people that I could and would use violence to achieve my aims. Consequently, my major fear since then is, that if I get angry enough, I could seriously hurt someone or even kill them. This constant worry has had a dramatic impact on my life and it's been an incredible drain on my mental health to resist such violent urges.

After this incident I headed down a path of using aggressive behaviour to achieve my goals. I became less sensitive to criticism and developed a superiority complex. If I did not trust a person, I did not care what they thought of me.

3. Incident with Commanding Officer

A later incident demonstrated to me that my technical skills could overcome my personality problems. Our Flight conducted a cordon and search operation on the village where significant VC activity was occurring. Our Air Field Defence Flight surrounded the village during the night and Vietnamese forces searched it after dawn. For some reason, the Commanding Officer of the Squadron, a bomber pilot, joined the operation. As he was only armed with a pistol and had no combat training, to my surprise I was instructed by the same person who made the comments above to look after him during the operation. He lay next to me with his pistol drawn but was shaking so much that I thought if we saw any action, he could shoot me! I convinced him to holster his weapon and trained him how to be my assistant on the machinegun, which I again was assigned to that night. My take on this incident was that in a tight situation my technical skills were enough to rely upon. If I performed well technically, I could even order a senior officer to do what I wanted!

There were many other incidents in Vietnam including a knife fight with a Mexican on the base a month or so after this incident and a serious bar fight in Malaya whilst on R&C in December 1970, which reinforced my new personality traits.

Consequently, for the rest of my tour I turned inward and vowed never to let people know that they could or had hurt me. I also started to drink and more importantly, after the knife fight and bar fight, I became fearful that I could indeed seriously harm or kill someone.

Indeed, this avoidance attitude acquired during my active service was based on the proposition that I was better than my peers and had little or no confidence in my superiors if I did not trust them. Furthermore, as stated, I objected to the notion that the RAAF hardly ever acknowledged the hard work and dangerous task we were undertaking. I do not recall any positive acknowledgement of our efforts from the Commanding Officer during my tour.

I could disregard my personality faults and just power on. To assist me, and as an excuse not to mix and drink, I started studying as a way forward and as another avoidance strategy. I would say I cannot mix or party because I was studying.

Return to Australia

On return to Australia I started to plan a way forward, seeking to change my employment in the belief that my personality failures would be left behind.

My last report as an Airfield Defence Guard demonstrated that although my plan for excellence was working my avoidance of personality problems persisted.

Today

It was only in 2018 that with the help of my Physiologist, Hannah Lupo, I reassessed the situation. Instead of the bloated opinion I had formed, the correct assessment was that my moral compass had not allowed me to injure a defenceless person and this had avoided the possible massacre of innocent people. However, even in 2020, I still believed in using aggressive behaviour to influence other people.

I am a work in progress.

MY NORMAL

Michelle Fraser
Veteran's Daughter

When you are young you only look at your parents with the purest of love. Our house was filled with love and there was never any doubt in my mind that my parents loved us and would do anything for us. We always had food, a comfy and cosy house and we rarely saw them fight. I can only recall one time from my childhood where Mum and Dad had a huge fight that resulted in Dad walking out the front door and slamming it behind him. I believe I was around five at the time and I remember crying and being so scared that my Dad was gone for good. Like most kids the thought of either of my parents ever leaving terrified me.

For the most part I can honestly say that my childhood was a happy one. However, whilst it was happy and we were never left wanting, there was always something lurking, a tenseness is the best way to describe it. There was love but with Dad, affection was often missing. I learnt very early on not to do certain things, a survival mechanism I guess, that would upset Dad: I learnt not to cry or not to be over-emotional (Dad hated the sound of us crying and would just get aggravated by my emotions); I learnt not to creep up beside his side of the bed when I had a bad dream or needed something in the middle of the night (if you startled him you might get flung across the room); I learnt not to tell him things that I know would upset him (he was tough, and I did not want to see someone else get hurt even if they had hurt me).

That was my normal – happy and content but walking around on egg shells.

Right up to the age of about 12 we had a "normal" military upbringing. Dad was in the Air Force and had served in Vietnam. He talked about the Air Force but never his time in the Vietnam. It wasn't until I was in my late 30s and 40s that I found out and am continuing to find out about Dad's time in Vietnam. We were posted every couple of years but looking back I considered our postings as lucky in military terms. We only ever lived in two cities; albeit moving between the two a couple of times. This helped with school as we always slotted right back in where we left off with usually the same group of friends who had more permanent upbringings.

Growing up, our Dad was always there for us on the weekend, our childhood was filled with bike rides, swimming trips to the pool or to the local swimming hole, trips to parks etc. He was present as a Dad.

We were also children of the 70s and 80s and if you misbehaved it usually brought a smack of some sort from the nearest adult available. This was the same with most of our friends so there was never any amount of physical violence that was excessive by the standards of the time. What I was afraid of however was the outburst of verbal rage that we would cop if we upset him. He would fly off the handle at the smallest thing that as children we did not understand. We learnt to call these rages as "tit drops". Up until our teenage years my older brother would cop the brunt of these, and I guess as the youngest child I learnt from his mistakes. I remember a time when he asked Dad for help with his long division homework – my brother (and let's face it, most of us when learning long division) just did not get it. He wasn't mathematically inclined and unfortunately for him he just did not get the concept behind the maths of long division. Because he did not get it Dad flew into a rage which resulted in my then 9-10-year-old brother being called every name under the sun, being told he was stupid and useless and then being smacked with his ruler. This rage seemed to go on forever and left my brother shaken and I learnt a very valuable lesson to never ask Dad for help with homework. From that day on I asked the teachers, friends, friends' parents, everyone else but Dad.

Dad was strict with us and as children we knew that there was to be no misbehaving. I recall a time when my brother and I misbehaved and disrespected mum. When Dad got home from work he flew into a rage that we had disrespected his wife, ordered us to pack our school bags with clothes, loaded us into the car and drove us off the military base, told us to get out of the car and never come home. I was terrified, especially after my brother told me not to follow him and I was on my own. Of course, Dad came and got us and we learnt a lesson from it. I was about eight at the time and it was dark.

When we were teenagers, Dad retired from the military after about 20 years' service and threw himself into civilian life and became a workaholic. My parents bought their first home and Dad went off to work as a civilian. Dad dropped out of our life a bit at this point. He was there but not there; he was consumed with work and we didn't really see him on the weekend. There was not much family time, time spent as a family was often at the dinner table or watching a TV show together during the week and like most teenagers my brother and I spent our weekends with friends. Our house was a welcoming house for our friends and my memories of those years were of friends sleeping over whenever they could. Parties at our house are still talked about 30 years on. My friends always knew they were welcome and could ask my parents for help any time they needed it.

The first time I learnt anything about Dad's time in Vietnam was through a teenage friend who told me what he had said to her after she interviewed him for a school project on the 60s. I remember feeling embarrassed that I knew nothing about what he experienced, ashamed that I had never asked and so distant from him that I felt I couldn't ask.

Neither Mum or Dad where big drinkers at home, there weren't any after-work beers cracked, wines with dinner or scotches on the rocks. However, Dad *was* a binge drinker where one was not enough and twenty was too many. His drinking was confined to Friday night drinks with the boys which often resulted in us waking up with dad passed out wrapped around the toilet on Saturday morning. Growing up, that was what I thought was the normal way to drink alcohol – go big or go home – after all as a teenager you only consumed alcohol at parties with mates and it was usually in a quantity that you would learn a valuable lesson from. Binge drinking was my normal.

Like most teenage girls this was also the time when I pushed my boundaries as much as I could. On reflection, I was a brat. My teenage outbursts were too much for my Dad, after all if he couldn't handle me getting upset as a child, you can only imagine how much a teenage girl's tantrums would aggravate him. We spent these years in constant conflict with each other. Time spent together always ended in an argument with Mum playing referee. No matter how I tried I just couldn't talk to him and rebelled constantly.

This continued well into my 20s and even 30s to an extent and so did my binge drinking. Stupidly at the time I was proud that I could drink a lot in one night and didn't see the impact it was having on my life and relationships. My friends on more than one occasion approached mum and dad with concerns over my drinking and at 21 my dad sat me down after one of my nights on the turps and told me he had bought a one-way bus ticket to Townsville for me. The ticket was booked for lunch time the next day. I had less than 24hrs to pack, was given $200 and told that I couldn't ask for any money and if I wanted to come home I had to make my own way back. We were living then in Darwin and the bus ride was 3 days.

After a small stint in Townsville living off the generosity of my Dad's cousin who I had never met, I decided to move to Mackay to where my Dad's sister lived. Time spent in Mackay under her guidance settled me down for a bit, however I landed a job in a local pub which still enabled me to continue with the binge drinking lifestyle I had grown used to and considered normal. It took Dad shattering his shoulder in a surfing accident and what little of my savings I had to get back home to Darwin a year later (on a bus again) with $50 to my name.

The partying and at times reckless lifestyle continued until my late 30s early 40s. Like most military children I felt it hard to settle in one place and bounced back and forth from Darwin to Brisbane every couple of years. To this day I still feel the itch to move every couple of years, whether it be a new flat around the corner or a new city, nowhere has ever felt like home. In between all this I managed to complete a university degree and establish a career hiding my weekend lifestyle from work colleagues and family. My lifestyle made it hard for me to maintain any sort of meaningful relationship, after all I was too busy partying on the weekends and busy working during the week to have a serious partner. A partner would also require me to be affectionate and open about my feelings which is something that I have struggled with my whole adult life. It's hard to open up to someone when you are raised in an environment where you are not allowed to show your emotions.

Throughout these years I didn't really speak much to my Dad. Mum was my go-to for things and chats. Dad didn't like speaking on the phone much back then so when we did, the conversations were few and far between and consisted of the very basics before he passed the phone to mum. For the most part it felt like he just was not interested in what was happening in my life and when we did discuss things like my career, the conversations often ended in an argument with him having zero patience with my opinions. Dad was well and truly a workaholic by this stage and whilst he would throw himself into work and any other social justice political cause that came along, he didn't have much time for us, especially not small talk with us. When we were together, the egg shells where still scattered around the floor around us.

During this time, I remember feeling jealous of my friends' relationships with their fathers. I would often compare my relationship with my dad to the ones my friends had with theirs. I found it bizarre but also craved their normal. The ease that they could talk to each other, have a quiet beer together after work, go to the football and genuinely want to be in each other's company. I wanted to have that sort of relationship with my Dad, but we just couldn't get there.

In my early 40s after waking up one day after a night of binge drinking accompanied by a blackout, I decided it was time to clean up my act. By this time, I had cut back on a lot the reckless behaviours of the past 20 years but had come to the realisation that I was, like my Dad a binge drinking alcoholic. I had also started to suffer from anxiety. It was around this time that my Dad also started to get professional help for his PTSD.

For me it all came to a head when my Dad, having started counselling, had started calling me more often and wanting to see me more. One day he rang to "inform" me that he was dropping mum off for dinner with me that night whilst he attended a veterans-only BBQ. I remember suffering a major anxiety attack at the thought that my mum was coming over for dinner, the anxiety was not so much that she was coming but that I only had one chicken schnitty defrosted. Later that afternoon I reached out to Dad for the first time that I can recall on an emotional level and asked for help as well.

Our family is a work in progress still. We have all made mistakes and been impacted by the last 50 years of my Dad's life, however we are all trying to work our way through it together. I rarely touch alcohol now and my Dad calls me and wants to speak to me daily. Our normal is still different from everyone else's normal. When I look at both my parents, living with PTSD and trauma is all they have ever known – both come from military families with their fathers serving in wars. It's generational, Dad's father was an alcoholic too, they only know a PTSD environment. It's their normal.

The best part of reaching this stage in our journey is that I now have my Dad back and am building a relationship with him like the ones I used to get jealous of with my friends. We are reliving in a way the best parts of my childhood. We have both taken up bike riding and hiking together. For the first time in my life I love being around my Dad and consider him my best mate.

SURVIVING AND THRIVING WITH PTSD

Jeanette Holland
(name in service: Jenny Holland-Bender)
WRANS Veteran

I left work late 2016. Well I decided to retire, I did not plan it, it just happened. A massive decision which was predominately led by lack of motivation to continue to work; ongoing severe mental health issues; non-existent private and social life; and more ongoing major physical health issues.

I then decided to move to Qld to be closer to my parents whom I hadn't really had a relationship with since I left home to join the Woman's Royal Australian Navy (WRANS) in 1976 at the age of 17.

Over the coming years, I became more aware that I always felt that there was something wrong (for want of a better term), which I now know was the fallout from major trauma. Some trauma I knew about and some was so very, very deep, too deep and sooo painful that it was locked down in a deep space and the key was thrown away permanently.

Like they say, when you stop, it all comes out . . . And after about 6-12 months living in the retirement phase of my life, thinking that I would kick back and everything would be rosy, well I could not have been more wrong.

I found the transitioning from Service life after 23yrs full time, 10yrs Active Reserve and 7yrs as a Defence Public Servant, difficult to say the least. Just the impact of change from Service to civilian life – the language, expectations, goal orientation, management – was all a massive upheaval and one that triggered those terrible feelings of inadequacy, self-worth, self-dignity, self-understanding, purpose and where and how I was expected to fit into this new environment.

I started volunteer work as an Advocate at my local RSL sub-branch and the Vietnam Veterans, thinking I could help other service veterans, and this would give me a purpose. It did initially but listening to all their traumatic stories triggered my own traumas, even though I didn't really know what they were.

I hit rock bottom, my world got smaller, I locked myself away in my house. Thank goodness for Freddy, my dachshund puppy, a life saver, otherwise I probably wouldn't have made it… He has helped me through many, many difficult, dark, low emotional times.

I was again diagnosed with a major health issue. A 2.5cm tumour was found by chance on my Pituitary Gland in December 2018. There was a real possibility of going blind (the second such experience for me). So, within 2 weeks I was in having major brain surgery and after a long recuperation period, things have now settled down, with annual MRI follow ups. I am only now realising the actual depth, magnitude and seriousness of this surgery. In the aftermath, the flood gates opened and lots of other physical health issues gushed out. My GP prompted me to look further so I finally put myself out there and saw a Psychologist and Psychiatrist. That was a massive turning point although it certainly took its time coming.

Over the years, like I said before, I knew I had something locked away in there – some trauma I was aware of (maybe didn't really want to acknowledge) but I did have an idea. I didn't realise the impact, and I didn't want to acknowledge any of it. Over the years I had sought help from both mainstream and alternative health modalities, and here I was doing it all over again again. Telling my story to someone I didn't know, and fearful that I would be judged and ultimately a report would go back to my supervisor, as did happen in the past. Great work, cause that's where it all lay: judgement, expectations and consequences for sharing my feelings and my story of what happened to me in the workplace.

THE TRAUMA

After many many tears, my own stubbornness and physical symptoms, some of which I will not disclose, but the most visual was that my throat would close over and I was literally unable to speak, so debilitating and frustrating it almost forced me not to speak at all, to keep it all locked away because it was way too painful. Eventually it had to come out and it all did come out.

I was raped in the early years of joining the WRANS. I also eventually accepted that I had suffered daily bullying, humiliation, sexual and personal harassment, by men mostly. This doesn't sound much but when you continually receive this form of abuse it does take its toll. This became accepted behaviour for me … this was 'deemed' as normal. Just get on with it. Don't know how many times I heard that.

My known trauma was when my husband committed suicide by hanging himself in the family bathroom in 1992 in Exmouth, North West Cape. My then 12yr old daughter and I found him and I tried to revive him with CPR which unfortunately didn't work. Whilst the initial support was there, again I was told 'to get on with it', only several weeks after his death. The impact of his death coupled with lack of official support impacted on my relationship with my daughter. Again, it may not seem like much but that treatment was abhorrent and the memory stays with me all these years later.

I have found it difficult to trust anyone which has had a huge impact on my family, personal and professional relationships. I am now on my own and have been for many years. This has had a major impact on my relationship with my daughter and my only grandson whom I have not seen or had contact with for many many years.

NOW

So after the last major tumour surgery, I thought this cannot be the rest of life: too scared to speak, too scared to be in life, too scared and angry angry angry. Angry at a lot of things that I was blaming myself for. With mainstream support, weekly appointments and travelling to India for a retreat, my understanding of myself and all those negative and debilitating beliefs came to the fore. Many many times I wanted to give up. But I didn't – this just couldn't be it for the rest of my life.

In early 2018 I was diagnosed with PTSD and a year later, I was given the opportunity to undertake the Trauma Recovery Program at the Cooinda Mental Health Unit on the Sunshine Coast Qld. Wow, I really had no idea what that would entail. It was 12 weeks, 3 days per week. Intensive, very intensive. I met like-people and started to realise I wasn't the only one feeling this way. All right, backgrounds and situations were different but same-same behaviours and thoughts.

With so many life-threatening illnesses, I subconsciously decided that I did not want to hide behind my overweightness anymore. I wanted to have the very best opportunity to forgive and understand myself. And I did. I have now lost over 30kgs which has had an impact physically and mentally. I now understand the why. That doesn't excuse the behaviour of those who labelled me or used me, especially those in supervisory or management positions.

I have found that Yoga, mindfulness, meditation, anything physical helps me on a day to day basis. I had been training to undertake Kokoda in July 2020, but unfortunately due to the virus situation this was cancelled.

I have tried many different modalities and still do. I have spent a lot of my own money on my mental and physical health because I am important, I have a choice and I am my best advocate. My PTSD and memories will not go away, and some days, triggers are worse than others. However, I am constantly reassured by my wonderful Psychologist that I will never go all the way back to where I was. I do think that my recovery can be quicker, now I have a lot of tools. But some days are still not so good.

I realised that I was living – literally living – in my head, thinking that I was the only one feeling that way and no one, no one would understand or have any idea how I was feeling. By living in my head, I was also trying to fix it, in my head. Well, let me tell you from experience, that didn't and doesn't work.

One of the biggest negative beliefs was that I had no self-worth, after many years of feeling like I had been living in an ongoing abusive relationship being in uniform. I realised I had no voice. You may well say *but you wore a uniform* and *how could that be*. Well it was a mask and one that I wore especially well.

So, 18 months later and with many, many different supports of spiritual, universal and conventional understandings, I am now managing day to day. Maintenance is the key. We were reminded at Cooinda, it's like tending your garden. Maintenance will make me grow and flourish. I also understand my own self-care. After years and years of supporting and giving to others, this was a difficult change, but I am now a priority. If I am no good, then how can I possibly help others?

Those who knew me back then or even at Cooinda, know that I really would never talk or speak, almost like a wall flower. So I listened, and gave in to my stubbornness and self-talk that it was all my fault.

I now have an online Facebook and Instagram blog, 'Warrior Queen Family', and a registered business, 'Warrior Queen'. This is a forum I created to have my own family of like-minded women by sharing my own stories and experiences via video. Sharing what worked and what didn't. I also have special guests sharing their own experiences and sharing their achievements and successes, whatever that looks like for them. I realised that now I have a voice, one that is important, one that counts and what I have to say matters. So I figured if I feel like this then there must be many others like me. There are. Another aspect of this is understanding our own achievements and successes because I found it difficult to acknowledge my own even though really there are so many. Again if I feel like this then there must be others the same. There are. My youngest Warrior Queen is 11yrs old and my oldest is 72yrs old. Age is absolutely no barrier.

I have designed and developed my business tag and logo. I have also designed and sell independently the 'Warrior Queen' active wear line of clothing.

This year I have been asked to share my story, how Warrior Queen came about, as a guest speaker with 'Women's Veteran Networking Association', a Podcast with international 'Community Cares' and another women's forum 'Women's Talking Stick'. I am extremely passionate about women speaking up and being heard and believe that this starts at an early age. What is more important is that everyone has a story and a story that should be told. We are all so very precious.

THE FUTURE

So what does the future hold? Well I am not sure. After years and years of regulated and mandated goal setting and massive professional expectations, I am revelling in the fact that I am now 'going with the flow' and trusting that life will show me and provide me with the opportunities when I am ready.

I can now say that I like myself. I know more about me than I have ever done. Joining the WRANS at such a young age, 17yrs, I didn't know who I was, what was important to me or how I should be . . . But now after lots and lots of work, I do like me and am finally understanding the true, authentic ME.

Thank you, Morgs for this difficult but wonderful opportunity. I must say it certainly was not easy to take my words and put them down on paper. This is only a small biopic of my life and experiences. This opportunity, combined with my videos on my Warrior Queen Family FB and Instagram page have been so liberating and my voice is getting louder and clearer.

Now it is one day at a time, literally one day at a time or one bite of the elephant at a time . . . I now have HOPE . . . And with HOPE comes a future and that is SOOOO exciting. HOPE I haven't had or felt for a long time.

I will manage my PTSD and not let my PTSD manage me.

Grateful Blessings, Thank you!!

Jeanette

GLOSSARY

A

AA	*Aurora Australis*. Australia's Antarctic icebreaker, also known as the Orange Roughy
AAD	Australian Antarctic Division
AAT	Administrative Appeals Tribunal
ABC	Australian Broadcasting Corporation
ACV	Armoured Command Vehicle
AD	Accidental discharge
ADF	Australian Defence Force
ADFA	Australian Defence Force Academy
ADG	Air Force Defence Guard
Admin	Administration
AIF	Australian Imperial Force
ANARE	Australian National Antarctic Research Expedition
Antarctic Apple or Melon	A red prefabricated fibreglass field hut made for Antarctic conditions. A melon is an elongated version of the apple.
ANZAC	Australian and New Zealand Army Corps
APC	Armoured Personnel Carrier
ATF	Australia Task Force

AWM	Australian War Memorial
AWOL	Absent without leave
AWS	Automatic Weather Station
B	
BA	Behavioural Activation
BA	Breathing Apparatus
Baywatch	Morning cleaning duties
BBC	British Broadcasting Corporation
B-52	A long-range, subsonic bomber built by Boeing
BBQ	Barbeque
Big Apple	New York City
Bivvy bag	A bivouac sack is an extremely small, lightweight waterproof shelter, and an alternative to traditional tent systems. The bag is zipped up over the user's head in order to shut out the elements completely.
Black box	Toilet box or can
BOM	Bureau of Meteorology
Booze	Alcoholic drink
C	
C	Celsius
Caddy	Cadillac motor car
CB	Confined to barracks
CB radio	Citizens band radio
CBT	Cognitive Behavioural Therapy
CBT-I	Cognitive Behavioural Therapy for Insomnia
CEO	Chief Executive Officer
Chopper	Helicopter
CIB	Criminal Investigation Branch
CMF	Citizen Military Force
CommCen	Communications Centre
Commos	Communists

CPAP	Continuous Positive Airways Pressure
CPR	Cardiopulmonary resuscitation
CSIRO	Commonwealth Scientific and Industrial Research Organisation
C3 C4 C5	Section of the neck area cervical vertebrae
D	
DART	Defence Abuse Response Taskforce
Dept	Department
DIL	Call sign – Delta India Lima
Dixie-basher	Kitchen hand
DJ	disc jockey/dee jay
DNA	deoxyribonucleic acid
Donga	Room
Down Under	Colloquial name for Australia
Duck	Lighter Amphibious Resupply Cargo vehicle
DVA	Department of Veterans' Affairs
E	
Electrolyser	A machine that makes hydrogen from electricity and water.
EW	Electronic Warfare
EnviroCom	Is an experienced environmental consultancy for education, research and training services to the public and private sectors
F	
FAC	Forward Aircraft Controller
FB	Facebook
FSB	Fire Support Base
Fuzzy Wuzzy Angels	The name given by Australian soldiers to Papua New Guinean war carriers who, during World War 2, were recruited to bring supplies up to the front and carry injured Australian troops down the Kokoda trail during the Kokoda Campaign

G

Giggle hat	Green light cotton hat
GMRF	Gallipoli Medical Research Foundation
GP	General Practitioner
GPS	Global Positioning System/Navigation device
Grunt	Infantry soldier
H	
Hagglunds	Swedish dual cab over-snow vehicle powered by turbo diesel engines driving four rubber tracks. It can carry four passengers in the front cab and can operate over most snow and ice terrain including sea ice and soft snow.
HMAS	Her (or His) Majesty's Australian Ship
I	
IED	Improvised explosive device
IHBT	Institute of Health Biomedical Innovation
IRT	Imagery Rehearsal Therapy
Isthmus	A narrow length of land at the northern end of Macquarie Island. The station is located on the northern end of the isthmus.
J	
Jolly	This is an Antarctic term for going off-station for pleasure rather than work.
JP	Justice of the Peace
K	
Kanga Pad	Kangaroo helicopter pad Nui Dat
Kiwi	A person from New Zealand
Km/hr	Kilometre per hour
KY-38	Secure Voice System encoder/decoder
L	
LARC	Lighter Amphibious Resupply Cargo vehicle

LIDAR	Light Detection and Ranging instrument that began detailed study of the middle atmosphere above Davis station in early 2001.
Lifer	Signed up for life
M	
Macca	Macquarie Island
Mack truck	Is an American truck
MET	Meteorology
mg	Milligram
MP	Member of Parliament
MP	Military Police
m	Meters
mm	Millimetre
MRI	Magnetic Resonance Imaging
N	
Nasho	National Serviceman
NCO	Non-Commissioned Officer
NSW	New South Wales
NVA	North Vietnamese Army
NZ	New Zealand
O	
OIC	Officer in Charge/Command
OSA	Obstructive Sleep Apnoea
Ozone-sondes	These sounded the atmosphere and fed back information such as pressure, temperature, humidity, wind direction and speed, before bursting at between 70,000-80,000 feet, usually about 80 minutes later. Also, registered ozone information.
P	
pH	Potential of hydrogen or power of hydrogen
PMR	Progressive Muscle Relaxation

PNG	Papua New Guinea
P & O	Peninsular and Oriental Steam Navigation Company
Possum	Nickname for the Bell Sioux light reconnaissance helicopter
PR	Public Relations
Provost	Military Police
PSA	Prostate-specific antigen
Psych	Psychiatrist
PTSD	Post Traumatic Stress Disorder
PX	Postal Exchange is a type of retail store featured on Military installations
Q	
Q Store	Quartermaster's Store
Qantas	Queensland and Northern Territory Aerial Services
QR	Queensland Rail
Quad bike	Honda Trx300 four-wheel
QUT	Queensland University of Technology
R	
RAAF	Royal Australian Air Force
RAP	Regimental Aid Post
RAR	Royal Australian Regiment
R&C	Rest and convalescence
R&R	Rest and recreation
RD	Regional Director
Red shed	Main accommodation building at Casey Station
RQR	Royal Queensland Regiment
RSL	Returned and Services League of Australia
RSM	Regimental Sergeant Major
RTA	Return to Australia

S

SAS	Special Air Service (Army)
SAS	Space and Atmospheric Sciences
SES	State Emergency Service
SF	Special Forces
Sigs	Royal Australian Corps of Signals
SigCen	Signal Centre
Sig Sqn	Signal Squadron
SLR	Self Loading Rifle
Slushie	Kitchen duties as scrubbing pots, scrubbing floors, peeling potatoes etc
SMO	Senior Medical Officer
SUDS	Subjective Units of Distress Scale

T

T	Trainee
TAFE	Technical and Further Education
TAW	Tactical Air Wing
T&PI	Totally and Permanently Incapacitated
TV	Television

U

UK	United Kingdom
US	United States
USA	United States of America
U3A	University of the Third Age
USAF	United States Air Force
Uc-dai-loi	Vietnamese for "Australian"

V

VB	Victoria Bitter (beer)
VC	Viet Cong/Vietnamese Communists
VD	Venereal disease
Vets	Veterans

VHF	Very high frequency
VVAA	Vietnam Veterans Association of Australia
VVCS	Vietnam Veterans' Counselling Service
V8	Voyage 8 of the season
W	
Wakey	the day you wake up and go home
WF2	Wind finding radar
WO	Warrant Officer
WRANS	Women's Royal Australian Naval Service
X	
X-rays	Painless test which produces images of structures in body especially bones using high energy electromagnetic waves
Y	
Z	
Zodiac	Inflatable boat

DISCLAIMER

Reading this story and some of the contents may trigger Post Traumatic Stress Disorder (PTSD) symptoms. If so, please contact the following Help Lines:

If you have served or are currently serving in the ADF, you and your family members can use:-

Open Arms
Veterans and Families Counselling (formerly
VVCS – Vietnam Veterans' Counselling Service)
1800 011 046 (24 hour) or **www.openarms.gov.au**

Lifeline
13 11 14 (24/7) or **www.lifeline.org.au**

Beyond Blue
1300 22 4636 or **www.beyondblue.org.au**

During my rehabilitation with my PTSD, I have often used the PTSD Coach Australia app and I have found it very beneficial:

> **PTSD Coach Australia** is an app that helps people understand and manage the symptoms of post-traumatic stress disorder, or PTSD. The App is based on the latest scientific understandings of PTSD, and was modified from the U.S. Department of Veterans' Affairs PTSD Coach app.
>
> PTSD Coach Australia has been designed for use by Australian veterans and serving Defence Force personnel. It contains:
>
> - Up-to-date information about PTSD and treatments for PTSD;
> - a range of symptom management tools and techniques;
> - a PTSD assessment – allowing users to measure the severity of their symptoms over time, plot the results, and email them to a health professional;
> - a scheduler that allows people to manage all their health appointments and activities;
> - information about where to find treatments and supports for PTSD in Australia– in the Defence health system, within the Department of Veterans' Affairs and in the community.

RedSix app

RedSix is aimed at helping lower the growing suicide rate amongst the Veteran Community.

www.redsix.com.au/what-is-redsix

I am a member of all the organisations below:

Mates4Mates

Here for those impacted by service

mates4mates.org

Soldier On

Support Veterans and their families

soldieron.org.au

Young Veterans:

Empowering the lives of Australia's heroes

www.youngveterans.com.au

DAVID W MORGAN CAREER TIMELINE

Born 4th March 1948 in South Yarra, Melbourne, Victoria.

Education/Schools:-

Somers State School Victoria.....1953

Mildura West State School Victoria.....1954-1955

Alice Springs State School Northern Territory.....1956

Balaklava State School South Australia.....1957 (3 months)

Echuca State School Victoria.....1957-1960

Echuca High School Victoria.....1961-1963

Caloundra High School Queensland.....1964-1966

Military service:-

Army No 123256

Rank: Private

<u>Citizen Military Forces</u>

Unit: 9 Royal Queensland Regiment

Service: 14 April 1966 to 10 July 1967 (1 year and 88 days)

Army No 123256

Rank: Corporal

Australia Regular Army

Service: 24 July 1967 to 23 July 1970 (3 years Nil days)

Royal Australian Corps of Signals

Units: 1st Recruit Training Battalion – Kapooka
School of Signals – Balcombe
139 Signal Squadron – Enoggera
104 Signal Squadron – Vietnam
4 Signal Regiment – Wacol
139 Signal Squadron – Enoggera

Army Trade: Operator Keyboard and Cipher

Service Overseas: 1 year and 1 day

Honours and awards

Australian Active Service Medal 1945-1975 with Vietnam clasp
Vietnam Medal
Vietnam Campaign Medal
Australian Defence Medal
Army Combat Badge
Returned from Active Service Badge

My career after Military service:-

1970 to 1971

9th August 70 to end December 71 Communication Cipher Operator with the Commonwealth Department of Supply, Melbourne, Victoria.

1972

Beginning January 72 to end June 1972 Communication Operator with the Bureau of Meteorology Darwin, Northern

Territory.

1972 to 1977

From July 72 to October 77 in the Regional Forecast Centre Brisbane as a Weather Assistant and APT Operator (Automatic Picture Transmission) Satellites.

During this period from February 75 to August 75, took Leave without pay and travelled across USA and Canada.

Married on the 5th of March 1977 to Debbie Leabeater.

1977 to 1978

24th October 1977 to October 1978 on the Bureau of Meteorology Technical Officer Meteorology Observer course at the Bureau Training Centre Melbourne, including 3 months on the job training at Eagle Farm Airport, Brisbane.

1978 to 1981

From October 78 to March 81 posted to the Meteorological Office at the Amberley Air Force Base in Queensland and including two temporary postings to Oakey Meteorological Office at the Army Aviation Base in Queensland.

1981 to 1982

From March 81 to March 82 posted to the Longreach Airport Meteorological Station Queensland.

1982 to 1984

Meteorology Qld Relief Office Pool, including postings: 2 months at Amberley, 2 months at Longreach, ten months in total at Rockhampton Airport, six months at Cairns Airport and the rest of the time at either Brisbane Airport or the Brisbane

Regional Forecast Centre.
Daughter Michelle born on 17th October 1983 at the Royal Brisbane Hospital.

1984 to 1987
From August 84 to December 87 posted to Charleville Airport Meteorological Station Queensland.
Son David born on 13th August 1985 at the Charleville Base Hospital.
Promoted to Technical Officer Grade 2 in April 1987.

1988 to 1993
From January 88 to April 93 posted to Gladstone Meteorological Station Queensland.
Promoted to Technical Officer Grade 3 – Officer in Charge, Gladstone Meteorological Station on 20th February 1992.
My mother Sybil Ornsby (Cookson) Morgan passed away on the 26th August 1992 at the Gladstone Base Hospital, age 83 years.

1993 to 2005
From April 93 to February 98 posted to Rockhampton Airport Meteorological Station Queensland as a Supervisor Technical Officer Grade 3.
After February 1998, I took temporary postings.
From March 1998 to September 1998, Officer in Charge, Giles Meteorological Station Western Australia.
From 2nd September 2001 to 22nd March 2002 ANARE Program – Australian National Antarctic Research Expeditions, Officer in Charge, Macquarie Island Meteorological Office.
From August 2002 to March 2004 ANARE Program –

Australian National Antarctic Research Expeditions.

From 22nd November 2002 to 4th December 2003, Davis Antarctica Base Meteorological Office.

Honours and awards

Australian Antarctic Service Medallion

From 17th February to 12th of March 2004 posted to Casey Antarctica Base Meteorological Office. After slipping on ice at Casey Base, I was medevaced back to Australia with severe head injuries. After medevac, I was on sick leave till retirement.

2005

After 33 years' service with the Bureau of Meteorology, I retired on 8th April on Doctors advice due to PTSD – Post Traumatic Stress Disorder.

Published Books

Title: *Ice Journey: A story of adventure, escape and salvation*

Published in 2010 by Big Sky Publishing Pty Ltd.

ISBN: 9780980658248 (paperback)

Title: *My Vietnam War: Scarred Forever*

Published in 2014 by Big Sky Publishing Pty Ltd.

ISBN: 9781922132772 (paperback) 9781922132789 (e-book)

MY LEGACY STORY

I have decided to share my Royalty payments to Legacy. Legacy is a great organisation which supports veterans' families.

My siblings and I were wards of Legacy. I don't know to this day how my mother and the family would have managed without that help. My wife Debbie was also helped by Legacy when her father died while she was young.

They shaped our lives by helping with our education, accommodation, and by purchasing push bikes, for instance, for my twin brother and me. All our legatees who were mostly war veterans became our surrogate fathers.

I became a legatee myself in Yeppoon in 2006 and 2007 but unfortunately, had to quit due to the effects of PTSD.